WOMEN ARE DYING, DEB

WOMEN ARE DYING, DEB

Inside America's Maternal Mental Health Crisis

EMILY E. JOHNSON, MHA

Published by: Emily E. Johnson
Printed in the United States of America
missionjustonemom@gmail.com

ISBN: 979-8-234-03150-1 (print)
ISBN: 979-8-234-03151-8 (ebook)

Cover Design by:
Danna Mathias Steele

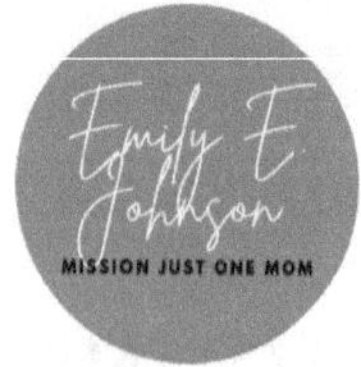

www.missionjustonemom.com

DISCLAIMER

This book is a memoir. It reflects the author's present recollections of experiences over time. The events, places, and conversations in this memoir have been recreated from memory. The chronology of some events has been compressed. When necessary, the names and identifying characteristics of individuals and places have been changed to maintain anonymity and protect their privacy.

This book is intended for informational and educational purposes only. It is not intended to provide medical advice, diagnosis, or treatment. The information contained herein should not be used as a substitute for consultation with a qualified physician or other licensed healthcare provider. Readers should not disregard or delay seeking professional medical advice based on information contained in this book. The author and publisher disclaim any liability for any loss, injury, or damage allegedly arising from the use or misuse of the information presented. The experiences described in this book reflect the author's personal experiences and opinions. They are not intended to represent medical advice or clinical recommendations. Individual outcomes may vary. Readers should consult their own healthcare providers regarding medical decisions.

CONTENTS

To Julian, who helped me change the world long before he ever even learned that the world needed changing. I am so grateful for you, my sweetest baby boy. Being your mom is the most amazing gift in the entire world.

Foreword

One in five women in the United States will experience a maternal mental health disorder such as postpartum depression or anxiety during pregnancy or in the year following childbirth. According to the Centers for Disease Control and Prevention (CDC), these conditions are both the leading complication of pregnancy *and* the leading cause of pregnancy-related death in our country. Yet despite growing public awareness, screening, diagnosis, and treatment for maternal mental health disorders are still not standardized and routine across the U.S. healthcare system.

I founded the Policy Center for Maternal Mental Health (originally known as "2020 Mom") in 2011 after my own experience with healthcare system failures through the birth of my first child and after losing a family member to suicide. These experiences, combined with 25 years of working for a large health insurer, shaped my understanding of the barriers that new mothers face to diagnosis and access to maternal mental healthcare: issues around payment structures, provider networks, insurance benefit design, and accountability measures.

We've seen meaningful progress over the past 15 years. Many states have expanded Medicaid coverage to one year postpartum, allowing new mothers to seek care when they need it. Many providers have implemented universal screening, and some have integrated mental healthcare into obstetric settings. Thousands of providers have been trained to recognize and treat these devastating, yet treatable, conditions.

We are proud of the progress that has been made, but we still have quite a way to go. Each year, my organization publishes state-by-state report cards evaluating maternal mental health performance across 20 evidence-based measures. In 2025, the national grade was a C-. Not a single state earned an A, and 19 states received Ds or Fs. Our 2025 "Risk and Resource Report" found that 84% of women of birthing age still live in areas with a shortage of maternal mental health providers.

Behind these statistics are real women—women like Emily. I met Emily in 2025 when she came to share her story at the Policy Center's annual Forum on Maternal Mental Health. As I listened to her speak, I heard echoes of countless other women's experiences: the delayed diagnosis, the dismissals by healthcare providers who should have known better, the desperate struggle to find appropriate care.

But Emily's story didn't end with her own recovery. As a healthcare administrator, Emily tried to initiate change within a local health system by documenting the gaps, proposing evidence-based solutions, and advocating for infrastructure-level improvements. The resistance she encountered in that process illustrates how difficult it is to make change without the right policy levers, payment incentives, and accountability measures in place.

The Policy Center exists to address this. We work to create conditions for change by conducting research, convening cross-sector stakeholders, and providing technical assistance to state agencies, hospital systems, and insurers. But policy change requires more than data and technical expertise. We also need stories that help decision-makers understand what these systemic failures actually mean for real women and families.

That is what Emily has given us in this book: a window into both the human cost of our healthcare failures and the institutional barriers that perpetuate them.

We can, and must, do better.

Joy Burkhard, MBA
Founder and Chief Executive Officer
Policy Center for Maternal Mental Health

Preface

My name is Emily. Until recently, I worked in healthcare business development. I have a bachelor's degree in economics and a master's degree in healthcare administration. My husband is a resident physician, and we've been together since he was a premed student in college, so I've been living, breathing, and talking about healthcare for most of my adult life.

When our son Julian was born a few years ago, I suffered from severe postpartum anxiety, obsessive-compulsive disorder (OCD), and depression. This caught me and my family completely by surprise, and we had no idea what was happening or what to do.

Spoiler alert: I had a pretty awful experience with the healthcare system when we first tried to get help. Then, at 15 days postpartum, I was admitted to a general inpatient psychiatric unit, which was scary, traumatic, and devastating.

But while I was in the hospital, my mom was able to find an incredible treatment program in our community. It was designed for pregnant and postpartum women suffering from the kind of severe symptoms I was experiencing. My journey to full recovery was a long one, but this program was the critical turning point and quite possibly the reason I survived.

Loss of hope is one of the most lethal pieces of postpartum depression, and that treatment program gave me and my family a reason to have hope in recovery. I truly cannot overstate the value of that.

One thing that I've found interesting since recovering from this experience is that few people seem comfortable seeing me as both a healthcare administrator and a woman with lived experience of severe postpartum depression and anxiety. I've been invited to share my patient story but then told to limit it to my traumatic story, not my observations or what I think needs to happen from my professional lens. And at work, I was allowed to speak about maternal mental health and the massive amounts of unmet demand in the market, but when I tied it into my personal experience, I was quickly dismissed for being "too close" to the topic.

However, what's most unique and valuable about my opinions on this topic is that I *am* both: I'm a healthcare administrator with an advanced degree from one of the strongest healthcare administration programs in the United States, *and* I'm a woman who was deemed, in writing, "high risk" for suicide two weeks after my beautiful, perfect baby was born. I feel that it's both my honor and my duty to share my entire perspective on this issue, so we can build a world where more women are able to access the kind of care they need to survive.

One of the first things I learned as I began to recover and look back on my illness journey was that I got unbelievably lucky to be where I was, when I was. Maternal mental health disorders are shockingly common, affecting an estimated one in five new mothers in the United States.[1] And we're not talking about just a little bit of sadness interrupting visions of newborn bliss; we're talking about serious mental health conditions that have devastating impacts on infant and maternal health.

Maternal mental health disorders are *the leading cause of maternal mortality* in the United States.[2] Yet an estimated 75% of women who suffer from maternal mental health disorders never receive treatment,[3] and the intensive treatment program I attended was one of only seven of its kind in the country at the time. This wasn't because it was a new and unproven concept or care model; there is, and has been for many years, data to demonstrate that these programs decrease depression and anxiety symptoms and increase levels of maternal functioning.[4,5]

So, that was one of the first things I wanted to understand. Given the prevalence of maternal mental health disorders and the impact they have on maternal morbidity and mortality, and given the research suggesting that specialized programs like the one I attended have a remarkable impact on symptoms, how on Earth do we have only a handful in the country?

The short answer is funding. I'd argue that the answer also has to do with the deeply ingrained and systemic undervaluation of women's health, but for now, let's focus on the more tangible answer: money. Intensive outpatient and partial hospitalization programs can be self-sustaining through insurance reimbursements, but they're costly to build and develop. This patient population has unique needs; it's not as simple as converting standard exam rooms into a program that thoughtfully supports both moms and babies. And that's even truer of inpatient units designed for this population.

At the same time, hospital margins have diminished over time, and many hospitals across the United States are currently struggling to break even.[6] Expansion aspirations aside, profit margins are what allow for new equipment, new technologies, and facility upgrades, so they're a big deal. Very few hospitals and health systems around the country are jumping up and down to use their limited capital dollars to build new programs that, at best, will be expected to break even, and at worst may end up costing them money to run.

When I started looking into the programs that exist today, I noticed a common theme. Many of them cite a specific benefactor or impetus for building their program. One such program is the Alexis Joy D'Achille Center for Perinatal Mental Health in Pennsylvania. After his wife Alexis died from postpartum depression, Steven D'Achille established a foundation that was able to build an incredible intensive outpatient program in her honor to ensure other women had more access to appropriate care.[7]

One of the things that has been deeply troubling to me is that healthcare leaders aren't learning from each other or proactively taking steps to close gaps in care where we know they exist. At the time I began my advocacy journey, the Alexis Joy D'Achille Center had been around for over a decade, yet *most states* in the U.S. still didn't have anything remotely like it.

One day, it hit me: at the rate we're going now, it's going to take a high-profile tragedy in every major city to generate support for building new programs like this and spreading this care model across the country. But I think that's bullshit. I think it's time that we say, "Enough is enough" and find a way to build the programs without waiting for a specific donor or executive leader in each health system to be personally impacted for this change to happen.

And that's why I tell my story.

Introduction

I used to be afraid to talk about what happened to me when my baby was born. It felt so ugly, so embarrassing, so shameful. On the surface, it felt much easier to simply describe it as "a really hard time," then move on. But inside, that approach wasn't easy at all. It allowed my guilt to fester and my worst memories to perch on the top shelf of my mind.

Slowly, with the help of a brilliant and compassionate therapist, I began to face my story. And as I did, something remarkable happened. I didn't just return to who I was, and how I was, pre-motherhood. I transformed into a stronger version of myself: more vocal, more protective, and less accepting of bureaucratic bullshit, particularly when said bullshit causes harm to moms and babies.

As a healthcare administrator, one thing I've known from the start of my advocacy journey is that failure is not an option. Too many women are dying from completely treatable illnesses, and too many children are growing up without the mother who should still be here.

Before my pregnancy, I'd sought a master's degree in my field for the purpose of improving healthcare and health outcomes in our country. When I stumbled upon the gargantuan problem of maternal mental health, which had some fairly obvious answers, I knew it was the opportunity I'd been looking for to improve the healthcare system. It was clear to me *from the moment I started to realize I might actually survive my illness* that on the other side, I was going to need to use my knowledge to improve the healthcare system.

When I initially started dreaming up the concept of this book, Part 1 was going to be about my personal story. Part 2 was then going to be about how I bravely shared my experience with executives at our health system and, together, how we took lived experience and turned it into meaningful, systemic change that improved the lives of thousands of women and saved the lives of some.

It was going to be a shining example for other healthcare systems and leaders about the promise of adopting a "just culture" and embracing an "improvement-first" mindset over the "deny and defend" mindset of the past.

It was going to be the start of a radical transformation in maternal mental health, one that would not only improve the lives of women in *my* community but also pave the way for other health systems in other communities to do the same.

But that's not what happened, so that's not what lies in the pages ahead.

The healthcare leaders did not respond with action and urgency, as I'd hoped; they responded with complacency and caution.

So, once I realized that my initial dream was not in the cards, I pivoted to plan B.

I started advocating on "the outside," amassing a large network of incredible maternal mental health advocates across the United States (and beyond!), all working toward the same goal: improved maternal care and reduced suffering from preventable and treatable conditions.

Alongside my own mother, who was filled with a similar level of fury about the experience we went through, I researched existing solutions and ways to expand those that are working well, of which there are many.

Everything you read here is plan B.

Part 1 is still about my own story, the good and the bad. Anytime you see something in italics, it's my inner monologue (or, as I sometimes call it, "the sneaky little bully in my head"). These lines represent real thoughts that I had, but they're often common myths and/or cognitive distortions related to my deteriorating mental health. Take anything this bully says with a grain, or a handful, of salt. You'll also see several "Hindsight notes," where I reflect on thoughts and experiences I had using the knowledge I've gained during my recovery and advocacy journey. These notes reflect my personal beliefs and opinions, though sometimes you'll see citations, because my beliefs and opinions are often evidence-based.

In addition to my own story, my book is now also about what happened when I initially tried to use my personal experience and my platform within healthcare to advocate for change, as well as what my mom and I learned as we began to pull back the hood on the larger issue of maternal mental healthcare.

Part 2 is my story of what it was like to advocate for change within a large nonprofit health system. I've used pseudonyms for both the organization and the individuals involved other than me. The point of this section is *not* to villainize the individuals or the particular health system involved in this saga. The point is, and has always been, to shine a light on a problem that's much bigger and more pervasive than my own story.

That's true about my postpartum anxiety and depression journey, and it's *also* true about my interactions with healthcare leaders following that journey. I know I'm not the first person who's tried to advocate for change within an imperfect system only to have that system shut them down, presumably in the name of risk mitigation. And I'm sure I won't be the last.

The point of Part 2 is to demonstrate just how hard it is to make change within large institutions today, and to show that many of today's healthcare leaders are failing to employ the "just culture" and "psychological safety" narrative they're teaching to young people entering the healthcare workforce.[8]

My ask of readers in this section of the book is to remember that these interactions aren't reflections of poor character or intentional harm. Rather, from my perspective, they're reflections of systems that aren't designed for change and individuals who've been taught to stay quiet and deny culpability whenever there's potential legal risk.

And finally, Part 3 of this book is an exploration of the gaping holes that exist in the healthcare infrastructure of the United States. These are holes that leave thousands of women and families suffering, and they're holes that don't need to exist. Throughout this section, I'll share my own opinions and research as well as insights from some of the incredible experts I've met along my advocacy journey.

I hope that, by the end, you'll see what I see: a massive opportunity for change. Change that won't just help women and families today but that will alter the course of history by going all the way *upstream* on mental health to the source of life itself: to the moms.

I'll even leave you with an action roadmap, so you'll know exactly what you can do depending on what role you play in the lives of perinatal people.

It will be far less satisfying than plan A, the alternative reality where I quietly and neatly addressed this issue from the "inside." But my hope is that you'll see that today's reality, one in which maternal mental health conditions are the leading cause of maternal mortality and specialized treatment exists only in an "underground network" sort of way, is now a choice. Furthermore, it's a choice that we can plausibly change within a single generation if we decide it's important enough to us. Most importantly, my hope is that you'll choose to act based on that knowledge.

This book is for moms (those who are currently struggling, as well as those who have already recovered) who need to see that it's the system that's broken, not them.

It's for the healthcare leaders who are interested in moving the needle on maternal mental health, and who aren't afraid of a young person's honest take on the current state of the industry.

This book is also for anyone who's concerned about the state of mental health in America, anyone who's curious about what's going on inside of the U.S. healthcare system, and anyone who wants a better future for our country.

PART 1

My Story

Content warning: This section contains vivid imagery of birth trauma and my subsequent battle with postpartum anxiety, OCD, and depression. I share details about troubling intrusive (as well as nonintrusive) thoughts, which might not be for everyone. You are more than welcome to skip to Part 2 if you'd prefer.

Disclaimer: Before I begin, I want to note that there are several different maternal mental health disorders, and that the symptoms of a given disorder can vary significantly across individuals (and across pregnancies, for that matter). My experiences may not reflect your experiences, your neighbor's, your sister's, or your hairdresser's.

I also want to acknowledge up-front that I am a white woman with tremendous amounts of privilege. I don't begin to know what it feels like to experience postpartum anxiety and depression in the context of poverty, social isolation, or racial bias.

But I do know what it feels like to "lose your mind" after having a baby and feel a tidal wave of guilt and confusion about it, and I know what it feels like to attempt to speak up about an important issue that has been stigmatized and under-resourced for a long, long time.

While there are *significant* disparities in the prevalence of maternal mental health disorders by race and socioeconomic status, it is also true that they can happen to anybody.

And they happened to me.

CHAPTER 1

Pregnancy

My pregnancy was, theoretically, medically unremarkable.

By that I mean I didn't have gestational diabetes, pre-eclampsia, or any other medical condition that put me or Julian at significant risk.

However, in another sense, it was medically the worst year I've ever had, by far. I had round-the-clock nausea and vomiting until well into my second trimester, followed by intermittent nausea and vomiting for the rest of the pregnancy. I quickly learned that "morning sickness" is a misnomer: for those who suffer from it, it's rarely limited to the morning.

Just three days into the start of the 24/7 nausea and vomiting, and weeks before my first official "prenatal" visit, I made a last-minute trip to the doctor's office saying, "Please help me; I can't live like this." I walked away from this visit with a prescription for Zofran and assurance that the misery I was experiencing was, indeed, "normal." A sign of a healthy pregnancy, in fact! Yay!

This was my first insight into how much physical misery directly related to our essential role in the continuation of our species women are expected to put up with while simply carrying on with regular life. I suppose I'd have learned this sooner if I were one of the millions of women who deal with severe menstrual cramps on a monthly basis, but thankfully, I'm not.

I quietly worked from home for the first week, because I hadn't yet learned how to distinguish "I feel like I'm going to puke" from "I'm actually about to puke," so I was afraid to drive on the highway for fear of throwing up and crashing. Eventually, I figured out this subtle but important difference and returned to my office with a supply of disposable puke bags on hand.

To help you understand what this early pregnancy experience felt like (especially for any men who might be reading this), and to ensure that I don't downplay the misery of this experience by simply looking back on it in hindsight, I'll share an entry from my journal during this time:

Late October, 2022

I'm 9 weeks and 1 day pregnant today and 3+ weeks into the nausea hellscape I entered in early October. Over the weekend, I briefly felt much more normal, so I thought there was a chance I was turning a corner. Then Monday came and it was back to the usual—wake up nauseous, medicate to the point of perpetual sleepiness, crawl through the workday, come home and crash on the couch in misery until it's time to go to bed. Usually with a nap thrown in somewhere, from which I usually awake nauseous and angry.

It's hard to get excited about being pregnant and becoming a parent when all I can think about all day long is what degree of terrible I feel. The nausea and vomiting make the pregnancy part seem very real, but somehow, in my mind, it hasn't made the idea of having a baby seem that real yet. I don't really feel ready for that—I'm not sure I have the instincts or the patience to be a really good mom. I feel guilty about that because my mom had all the patience in the world and always seemed to know what she was doing. I feel like I should be able to give that to my kids as well, but I don't know if that's in the cards. Thank goodness she lives so close, so my child can experience her caregiving skills the way I did as a child.

I haven't figured out when to tell my parents or Alex's yet, and I'm a little nervous for what that will be like. I'm sure they'll all be happy, but I think it might be overwhelming. For one, they'll probably all be completely shocked, which is both fun but also a little bit exhausting because it's a reminder that maybe you chose the uphill/questionable choice (which is why people didn't see it coming).

Oh, and it's Alex's birthday. We did a few fun things like order pizza and eat chocolate chip cookies, but I feel bad that I still complained to him a ton and didn't help with things like Howie care. It's really hard to believe that next year on his birthday we'll have a 5-month-old! I wonder if that will be easier or harder than what we're currently living through.

Sorry this was all so negative—I've been having a hard time seeing the happy side of life these days given my physical state. Hopefully, by the next time I write, I'll be in a different stage of this crazy journey.

Em

It's hard to comprehend how awful this severe nausea experience is unless you've lived it. And, to make matters more complicated, working women suffering from severe first-trimester pregnancy symptoms are faced with a dou-ble-edged sword when it comes to disclosure:

> *Should I share my pregnancy news with my boss early, so that I can (maybe) get accommodations but risk being treated differently for longer due to my pregnancy and shar-ing the news during the window when the risk of miscar-riage is still high? Or should I keep the news safely to myself but risk my boss coming to the conclusion that my change in behavior and energy level is just a reflection of my being lazy and/or less competent than I once appeared?*

I chose somewhere in the middle: I kept it to myself for as long as I could, riding on my previously built reputation for being an intelligent hard worker. Then, I shared the news with my boss about a month into the 24/7 nausea, when I really started to worry whether people were starting to see me as lazy, low energy, and less ambitious than I once was.

My boss was kind, but they didn't proactively offer any ac-commodations. I said that I'd been struggling with nausea and food aversions. Perhaps I should have been more vocal about exactly what would be helpful, but I was already nervous about the impact pregnancy would have on people's perception of me, and I was afraid to make it worse by asking for special treatment.

They must not have understood what my limitations were, because they proceeded to organize a mandatory team lunch for the next week. I was terrified. I hadn't eaten much besides Jell-O and Goldfish for the last four weeks, so I wasn't sure how on Earth I was going to make it through a catered team lunch.

Looking back, my anxiety was present from the very beginning of my pregnancy.

I found an online calculator of the chance of miscarriage by day, and I updated it each morning for the small amount of relief I'd feel when I saw the number tick down ever so slightly. Sure, I probably knew that it wasn't "normal," but it took less than a minute out of my day, so I didn't think much of it.

You have to reach the level of functional impairment for anxiety to be a big deal, right?

Later in my pregnancy, I started having panic attacks. These weren't entirely new for me; I used to have an intense fear of flying that would sometimes result in mid-flight panic attacks. But midway through my pregnancy, I began having panic attacks out of nowhere, which was unusual for me.

One night, I was home alone while my husband was at work (a common scenario, as he works in medicine). Suddenly, I was struck with intense fear and a sense of impending doom. I'd been planning to relax and take a bath, but that was now out of the question, because I thought I might somehow die if I did that.

I didn't know what to do, but I didn't want to be alone, so I called my mom. I told her I was feeling anxious and just wanted to be on the phone, so she happily chatted with me for half an hour. At one point, I had to mute my end of the conversation and just listen to her voice, because the anxiety was so intense that it was giving me diarrhea.

Eventually, the feeling passed, and I tried to just put that odd, awful experience behind me.

During one of my next prenatal appointments, I shared with my OB that I was having more anxiety than usual, in the form of panic attacks. She offered to start me on antidepressants. I declined, stating that since my issue (I thought) was primarily with episodic anxiety, I would prefer some sort of as-needed medication as opposed to a daily medication.

The unspoken part of this conversation was that I assumed it was always best to avoid medication during pregnancy whenever possible.

I have never taken psychiatric medications before. Why would I start now?

Hindsight note: Because the risks of untreated anxiety are higher than the risks of taking well-studied antidepressants during pregnancy.[9,10]

We settled on an ad-hoc antihistamine called hydroxyzine. We didn't discuss the concept of therapy. In retrospect, I can't help but wonder how many things would have been different if I'd started looking for perinatal therapy at this point in my journey instead of several months later, when I had a one-week-old baby at home and was running on fumes.

Throughout my pregnancy, there were a few other foreshadowings of my later mental health battles.

One was the number of times I sought urgent or emergent care. I was seen in Labor and Delivery (L&D) triage three times: once for a (gentle) slip on ice while walking my dog, once for gas pains that I mistook for something far more severe, and once for some random pain in my stomach toward the end of my pregnancy that felt "like a bad bruise."

I also made a last-minute same-day appointment one day because I was worried I hadn't felt the prerequisite number of kicks in a given time period; I was seen in urgent care on another occasion because I had a pilonidal cyst, and I was worried about whether it would be an infection risk during delivery.

To be clear, none of these on their own are wrong, and I would never suggest that somebody with concerns about their pregnancy avoid seeking care. However, they do reveal a pattern of deep concerns that all ended up being nothing out of the ordinary. This should have been a clue about the escalating levels of anxiety I was experiencing, if anyone had been watching.

The other noteworthy foreshadowing was my very first conscious "intrusive thought." Intrusive thoughts are common and happen all the time.[11] Often, they're innocuous or absurd, so we don't pay much attention to them. But during the perinatal period, intrusive thoughts can crop up around harm coming to the baby, and suddenly, the random thoughts can feel more difficult to ignore.

My husband and I were touring a house, because we'd recently come to the realization that trying to raise a baby in our one-bedroom condo along with our high-energy husky mix would likely be a nightmare. As we walked around the basement of this house, the realtor pointed out a crawl space. Just then, a thought popped into my mind, with no warning:

What if I kill the baby and hide him in the crawl space?

Followed very, very quickly by:

Holy shit. What kind of sick monster thinks something like that? What if anyone finds out that I had a thought like that? They'll lock me up and/or take my baby away. Better keep that to myself.

I, like everyone, had experienced intrusive thoughts before, but I couldn't remember ever having any that were this violent or specific. I was *horrified* that my brain was capable of producing that thought, and I didn't know how to make sense of it. I certainly didn't jump right to, "Oh, here's yet another normal, but extremely uncomfortable, pregnancy symptom."

So, I'll pause and issue an invitation to anyone who's recently experienced an unexpected, disturbing intrusive thought: one that you're horrified of and would never want to have actually happen. You may chalk it up as just another normal, though extremely uncomfortable, pregnancy symptom,[12] but consider mentioning it to your doctor and/or therapist so they can help you manage your symptoms.

———

As my mental health symptoms escalated, my physical symptoms continued kicking my butt too. I had it all: nausea, vomiting, food aversions, debilitating pubic symphysis pain, constipation, hemorrhoids, heartburn, fatigue. A tough blow psychologically for someone who was raised by a mother of four who's forever claimed that pregnancy and delivery were always a breeze for her.

What if the degree to which you can handle, or enjoy, pregnancy is an indicator of how good of a parent you'll be?

Hindsight note: It's not.

Then, in my last few months of pregnancy, I got COVID-19, went through a particularly rough patch of seasonal allergies, and then got another nasty respiratory bug that landed me on the couch with a fever and no energy.

I have a vivid memory of calling my sister in tears during that time, asking her how I was going to be able to care for a newborn in just a few weeks (or less). I was so completely and utterly depleted. Not just from my acute illness, but from the cumulative experience of the previous nine months.

CHAPTER 2

Warning Signs Left, Right, and Sideways

Labor

I know this will attract my fair share of critics, so I'll say it here first and own it: I chose to have an elective induction.

On top of being physically miserable, I was terrified of something going wrong, and I saw each passing day as an opportunity for my body to turn on me and fail my baby somehow.

In a rather unfortunate turn of events, when I was maybe a month shy of my due date, I was in the office when someone got the news that a friend of theirs had just had an unexpected full-term stillbirth. New fear level unlocked.

I'd already been considering an induction for scheduling purposes related to my husband's medical training (more on that another time!), but this story pretty much solidified it.

The sooner I can get this baby out of my body so that I'm not the only one responsible for his survival, the better.

By the time I went in for my induction, I was ready to be done with pregnancy. I (naively) thought that from a personal health perspective, I was nearing the finish line and all I needed to do was get through labor and delivery. I knew that caring for a newborn would be intense and extremely challenging, but at least I would physically and mentally feel much better, right?

The day of my scheduled induction, we were running late. We were, of all things, returning a baby gate that we no longer needed, because we'd made a last-minute decision to move a few weeks before the baby came.

Hindsight note: I do not recommend this! Stressful life events, such as moving, are a known risk factor for postpartum mood disorders.

That errand took longer than anticipated. I started getting really irritated with my husband: "We're going to be late! We're going to be late on the single most important day of our lives so far!" I was livid, embarrassed, and feeling guilty for inconveniencing the hospital and OB teams.

We can't even get to the hospital on time. What does this say about our ability to be good parents?

Hindsight note: Nothing. Literally nothing.

We checked in, and I apologized profusely for our tardiness. I was reassured by a kind nurse that it was fine.

Before my epidural, I spent a lot of time walking the halls with my husband. At one point, we passed a computer screen where someone had left a training module of some sort up. The content on the screen read (and I wish I were making this up, but I'm not), "How to use a morgue bag."

I pointed it out to my husband, genuinely spooked but also able to recognize the complete absurdity of the situation. I asked him (only partially kidding) if this was a sign that they were getting ready for my inevitable demise. Jokes aside, this hit directly on—and validated, to an extent—one of my biggest fears: dying in childbirth.

Morgue bag incident aside, my first evening of labor was uneventful. My husband and I binge-watched several episodes of *Queen Charlotte*, walked the halls, and ate restaurant-quality, custom-ordered stir fry from the hospital menu.

———

Things started deteriorating overnight, when the reality set in that I was unlikely to get a full night's sleep again for a long, long, long time. I was barely dilated and not much was happening, but a nurse would come in what felt like every 30 minutes to adjust the fetal monitor.

Oh my God, they're not planning to let me sleep. And everyone knows you don't really get to sleep once the baby comes. I'll never sleep again.

Eventually, I snapped[i] and asked the nurse to please let me get some sleep, even if it meant not having a perfect read on the baby the whole time.

---

i   By this, I mean I had the audacity to make a reasonable request; as a lifelong people pleaser, this felt like snapping.

She seemed surprised, but agreed. "So, should I put a note in your chart to not come back for a few hours?" she asked me, probably shortly after midnight. "Yes, thank you," I responded, too ashamed to tell her that I was actually hoping for nobody to disturb me until at least 6 or 7 a.m.

What kind of mom prioritizes her sleep over certainty about the health of her baby?

Hindsight note: The kind of mom who's smart enough to realize that labor is a marathon and that she would need her energy to push the baby out and care for him afterward. That's who.

The next day, things were progressing slowly, so the team began to escalate the interventions, including things like inserting a Foley balloon.[ii]

I don't feel ready, but I was the one who decided to come in for an induction. I'm taking up their time and space. It would be rude of me to ask to wait longer before escalating the interventions; I'm already taking too long.

I let out an actual scream when they removed the first balloon. Oops: my intense pain was a reflection of the fact that they'd removed the balloon too soon. So, they inserted a second one.

I opted to wait for a long time before deciding on an epidural, not sure yet whether I wanted one. I wasn't opposed to using medications for pain control, but I (accurately, as you'll see) predicted that being bed-bound and unable to completely

---

ii   A Foley catheter balloon is a tool that can be used to manually dilate (aka open) your cervix.

feel my lower half would be anxiety-producing for me. I wanted to at least delay that for as long as possible.

At the 24-hour mark, things were still progressing very slowly, so they recommended that they break my water to move things along. I agreed, but I quickly regretted it. Seemingly instantaneously, my contraction pain went from a manageable four or five to a nauseating nine.

At this point, I demanded an epidural, sure that I couldn't possibly survive pain like that for much longer. Fortunately, the anesthesiologist arrived fairly quickly and, thankfully, administered my epidural without any issues.

With the epidural, my physical pain evaporated, but it was soon replaced by a mental pain that was just as torturous. It felt like a several-hour panic attack: my heart was racing, I was overcome with terror about everything that was happening, and I could no longer concentrate on anything other than the fear I was feeling. I started shaking from the medications, and this sent my anxiety even higher, to the point where I was literally pleading for escape.

I called my mom, who was out to dinner, and asked if she would come to the hospital right away. At this point, the only thing I could think or talk about was how anxious I was, and I didn't want to keep burdening my husband with hearing that on loop. I also wanted him to have a chance to go find some food, but given the state I was in, I wasn't comfortable with him leaving me alone.

Hindsight note: My husband is amazing. Marrying him is the best choice I've ever made. He's a wonderful human being, and I love him dearly. And... his comfort and nutrition status should *not* have been one of my top concerns while I was enduring the worst physical and mental pain of my life delivering *our* child.

My mom came right away, and the tears began flowing the instant I saw her. "I can't do this, Mom," I said. "I can't do it. I'm so tired. I want to be done," I kept repeating.

My mom, as you'll come to see later in this book, is a saint. She'll panic over the strangest things ("Who put a wooden spoon in the dishwasher? Those are hand-wash only!!! [MY DAD'S NAME HERE]!!!"), but she can stay *remarkably* calm and comforting during a crisis. She held my hand, held on to me, and talked to me for hours.

Each time the team came to check my status, I assumed we were close, only to hit a tsunami of frustration and panic when they announced yet again that I was no further dilated than the last time.

I began stating more seriously to anyone who would listen that "I wanted to be done." My husband started to get worried, knowing that a C-section, while technically a way to grant this wish, would not necessarily be an easier route—far from it. Around midnight, we agreed that I would try to get some sleep, and that we would revisit the C-section conversation in the morning. My mom left, promising that she'd be back first thing the next day.

Shortly after my mom left, a young nurse came in and suggested a new position for me to try. "It may seem silly, but I've seen it work for a lot of other moms," she told me as she helped me maneuver into position with a yellow, peanut-shaped exercise ball.

And just like that, after over 30 hours of labor, things started moving, and moving fast.

I'll never know whether it was the new position my nurse recommended or just a coincidence, but finally, things were happening (though either way, I'm paying more attention to the nurses next time!). The OB team thought it was too soon, but given how I was feeling, they did a check "just in case."

After she was finished, the doctor who came to check me said, "Alright Emily, here's the deal."

I braced myself for disappointment, given the experience I'd had with every other cervical check thus far.

"You're 10 centimeters dilated, and it's time. Your baby is almost here. Give me one minute to go get the rest of the team."

I could hardly believe it. My mind relaxed for the first time in over eight hours, and I broke out into a huge smile. I was about to meet my baby. I was about to be done.

Delivery

My sweet baby Julian was finally born at 1:26 a.m.

When he arrived, I had about 30 seconds of the intense, all-consuming feeling of love that you hear about in movies. After 20 minutes of pushing with every ounce of strength I had, a wet, screaming, baby was placed on my chest, and I felt a rush of emotions that's impossible to describe.

I did it! I grew a whole human being, and after worrying about him daily for nine months and being in labor for over 30 hours, I delivered him safely. He was perfect.

But within minutes of Julian being placed on my chest, I was overcome with the most powerful need for sleep I've ever felt. I had to fight intensely to keep my eyes open. The care team tried to help me breastfeed my son, but they quickly decided it wasn't safe because I couldn't hold him without dozing off.

Guilt descended upon me quickly.

A good mom would want to stay awake to meet and feed her baby. I can't keep my eyes open. Either I'm a bad mom, or I must be dying.

The care team was speaking calmly and in hushed tones, but I could tell that things weren't going well. They were trying several different things, of increasing intensity, to stop my bleeding.

"Am I dying?" I quietly asked one of the staff members.

I still can't tell you whether it was the OB-GYN attending or a nursing student; it was just someone taking care of me who I figured probably knew the answer. My anxiety had mostly dissipated, and now I was just tired and deeply sad, thinking that I might not have the opportunity to watch my beautiful baby boy grow up.

At that moment, I just wanted to know.

But before I could comprehend the response, I slipped into a deep sleep.

My next memory is of being wheeled to the postpartum unit several hours later, semiconscious. It was like a little parade; there were people applauding me as I was wheeled past. But I didn't feel like celebrating. I was disoriented, I had blurry vision, and I had no idea where my baby was.

When we got to the postpartum room at about 5 a.m., Alex and I sent a message to our immediate family sharing that the baby had been born, that both of us were okay, and that we were going to try to get some rest.

"Name? Stats?" my brother-in-law responded.

I felt numb, and also angry about his questions. It was as if what I'd just accomplished wasn't enough on its own, and I was already behind on letting them know "the important things" such as how much Julian weighed (and, for the record, I had no idea). I slipped back into sleep.

I woke up again a few hours later, and I saw my husband and my baby both sleeping peacefully.

The reality that I was now responsible for this teeny tiny human started to set in. But I'd lost nearly two liters of blood, and I had barely enough energy to stand up, let alone care for another person.

I began to panic, and I told my husband that he needed to get up because I couldn't "do this" (be awake) alone. He firmly declined, explaining to me that he'd been awake the whole time doctors were working on me (stockpiling some trauma of his own). The time we got to the postpartum room was the first time in over 24 hours that he'd been able to sleep.

I hadn't realized that.

So, I let him go back to sleep, though I was now buzzing with anxiety and confusion.

I remember calling my sister that morning and admitting to her, racked with guilt, that I wanted nothing to do with caring for my son. My sister, who'd also experienced severe complications after the birth of her first child, said, "Oh, don't worry, I get it. I had no interest in holding [my niece] the day she was born."

Phew. Maybe this isn't a sign that I'm a terrible mom with no maternal instincts. Sure feels like it is, though.

That whole day, I remember feeling an intense urge to get up and walk around, though I was still very weak from the blood loss I'd experienced during and after delivery.[iii] It was late May, and the L&D unit had a beautiful courtyard attached to it. I desperately wanted to spend some time outside, but I wasn't allowed to go anywhere alone given my fall risk status.

---

iii   My hemoglobin level was around 7 g/dL. For context, the normal range for women is 12.0–15.5 g/dL. For pregnant adult women, the range is about 10.5–15.0 g/dL. Hemoglobin levels below 6.5 g/dL are generally considered life-threatening.

It dawned on me that I couldn't just ask my husband to come with me. We now had a baby that we were responsible for and couldn't just leave behind.

Oh my God. I'm trapped.

———

At some point that day, my OB visited and I shared how anxious I had been over the last week and throughout my long delivery. This time, when she offered to start me on an antidepressant, I quickly accepted, because I knew something felt very off. She also sent a social worker in to see me, who asked if I was in need of resources such as baby care items (I was not), gave me a packet of information about postpartum depression, and instructed me on who to call if I noticed (the typical) signs, such as intense sadness or frequent crying spells.

Breastfeeding

Going into delivery, I would've told you I was agnostic about breastfeeding.

Of course we'll try, but I'm open to using formula if it doesn't work for us. We'll see.

It wasn't until I was trying to breastfeed and failing that I realized how deeply I *did* care about breastfeeding, and how much I'd internalized the widely used mantra "breast is best."

Breastfeeding didn't come naturally to me or to Julian. I worked closely with the nurses and the lactation consultants in the hospital, but he struggled to latch, and when he did, he'd fall asleep 30 seconds later and we'd need to start over again.

Wow, I'm terrible at this. This is probably my fault somehow.

I found the process extraordinarily frustrating, especially because I was still so tired and each attempt took a lot out of me. I quickly came to resent it, and I felt a sense of dread each time the nurses showed up to try again—along with corresponding guilt *about* the dread I was feeling.

But at no point did this process feel even remotely optional.

If breastmilk is best for my baby, voluntarily choosing to stop offering that to him would make me a bad mom, right?

Hindsight note: No. The single most important thing for a baby is a healthy caretaker. Whatever it takes for the caretaker to be well is the best thing for the baby.[13]

So, despite our mutual frustration with the process and the amount of extra anxiety it caused me, I pressed on, determined to make it work.

Gearing Up to Go Home

The night before we were discharged home, we had Julian spend time in the hospital nursery so that we could get some sleep.

The only problem was, I *wasn't* able to sleep.

My mind was racing, and none of the tools I normally used to quiet my brain if needed (like listening to a podcast) worked. That night, I lay there awake, thinking and worrying about how important it was for me to get some sleep but completely unable to do so.

When the nurse came in the next morning and asked me if I'd gotten some good sleep, I told her honestly, "Not really.

I think it was because I was putting too much pressure on myself to sleep, so I couldn't? I'm not sure."

She paused, just long enough for me to realize that perhaps that wasn't everyone's experience.

"Oh, I'm sorry to hear that," she responded.

Hindsight note: Not being able to sleep while your baby sleeps when you're tired and sleep deprived is a common and significant warning sign of anxiety and/or depression.[14]

Later that morning, a car seat safety lady came into our room to do a demonstration of how to properly put Julian in the seat, tighten the straps, and know when to move the straps to the next setting.

I couldn't understand the lesson about when to move the straps for the life of me. This caused instant frustration, panic, and anger, because it made me feel stupid—and, worse, incompetent as a parent.

"I don't get it. Can you explain it again?" I asked.

She did. Still nothing.

"I'm too overwhelmed to learn right now," I said. "Show my husband, and he'll teach me another time."

"Okay," she said cheerfully. "That's okay; there's a lot of new information coming at you right now."

She proceeded to show just my husband.

Hindsight note: Not having the capacity to learn how to strap a child into a car seat is not a normal level of overwhelm. (No citation. I'm just reasonably certain this is a fair statement.)

Before she left, she said, "Oh, and I saw that you have a mirror hanging on one of the back passenger seats. You'll need to remove that before you leave. Anything other than the car seat poses a risk to your baby's safety."

Okay, noted. How did I not realize that? I should've known. She must think I'm careless. How am I going to keep my baby safe at home once we no longer have all of these people available to point out all of the mistakes we're already making?

Our First Day Home

I don't remember much about our first day home, but I remember not wanting my mom to leave. My husband thought we should have her go home overnight, but I insisted that we should at least have her stay downstairs on our couch so she could be there "just in case." We handled all of the overnight feedings, obsessed with the concept of doing everything ourselves, as if that would somehow signal that we were good parents.

The first time we tried to breastfeed in the middle of the night, my husband instantly vetoed the process. As usual, it wasn't clicking right away, so I was getting frustrated—as was Julian.

"We are not doing this," my husband said, getting out the pumped colostrum and a syringe.

My shame and guilt amplified. I felt that I was failing at a task that I *should* be able to master, one that so many other women seemed to do effortlessly.

I'm making both my baby and my husband miserable.

Maternal Danger Signs

While some of my ever-growing anxiety was misplaced, some of it was based on very real threats to life.

When I was discharged from the hospital, I was told that clots larger than a quarter were something to watch out for, among other things. The precise term used in my after-visit summary was that large clots were a "maternal danger sign." Or, in anxiety-speak, large clots were one of the "signs you might die."

The day after we got home, I stood up after using the bathroom and felt something huge and slimy fall from my body.

I'd passed a clot about the size of a playing card. My eyes filled with tears; panic and anxiety set in immediately. I had flashbacks to all of the headlines and statistics I'd seen about how many women die from pregnancy complications *after* being discharged from the hospital.

This could be it.

From the bathroom, I called my clinic's 24/7 nurse line. I shared what had just happened. The nurse on the other end sounded worried, which increased my anxiety 10-fold. She advised me to go to the emergency room (ER) immediately, so my husband and I packed up as fast as possible and returned to the hospital, bringing three-day-old Julian with us.

What if he catches some sort of respiratory disease from being in the ER? He's so little; he could die. Which is worse: bringing your days-old child to the ER and exposing him to germs, or leaving him at home with a grandparent but no food source other than formula?

> **Hindsight note:** It's time to start dismantling the implicit association between formula and poison that we've accidentally instilled in new moms, largely through the well-intentioned but off-the-rails "breast is best" movement. Leaving Julian at home with my parents (and formula) would have been safer for both me and my baby. But instead, I chose to bring him with me, so I could keep trying to breastfeed and/or offer him exclusively pumped milk.

When we got to the ER, there was confusion about where I should go. The young male nurse doing my initial intake told me that, given how recently I'd given birth, I shouldn't be in the ER but should be back at L&D triage.

This was music to my ears, because I was much more comfortable with L&D triage (which, as you know, I'd visited frequently) than with the ER.

"Yes, I'd like to go there, but the nurse line told me to come here. But I would really prefer to go back to L&D, if that's okay."

He called L&D, and they responded that no, they did *not* take postpartum patients, so I needed to stay in the ER.

Meanwhile, several staff members in the ER, including this young male nurse, asked me, "So, when did the bleeding start?" This instantly signaled to me that they knew very little about vaginal childbirth.[iv]

Cue the flashbacks again to headlines about women being discharged from ERs after birth, only to die at home.

Nobody knows what to do with me. They have no familiarity with childbirth. The clock is ticking. I can't afford to lose much more blood. I could die.

---

iv   Vaginal bleeding after childbirth, called lochia, is normal (and expected), and typically lasts for several weeks.

They brought me to a room, and right away, I requested a breast pump. In our rush to get back to the hospital, we didn't remember to pack ours.

Just the day before, I'd been using a hospital-grade pump at the very same hospital, so I naively assumed that the same amenity would be available to me this time.

Newborns have to eat every two to three hours, but I had to ask repeatedly, and it took several hours to get access to a pump. One of the times I checked in about it, panic escalating about the fear of starving my brand-new baby, a young staff member (I have no idea what her role was) asked me callously, "Can't you just breastfeed him?"

I shook my head and started crying.

"Okay, well, how about formula? I know we have some of that," she offered.

"No, I just really want a breast pump," I responded tearfully, the overwhelm evident in my voice. "I know you have them here. I was using one two days ago."

<hr>

Someone told me they would need to do an internal (vaginal) ultrasound to determine how much blood was in my uterus.

"Are you sure? I just gave birth vaginally a few days ago. I thought—"

Yes, they were sure, they responded.

I was wheeled down the hall to the ultrasound room, where the technician proceeded to do an external (abdominal) ultrasound.

"Are we doing an internal ultrasound too?" I asked, in a desperate attempt to self-advocate given my fear of being a maternal mortality statistic. "They said they were sure that I need that."

"No," the technician laughed. "You just gave birth a few days ago! We'll only do that if absolutely necessary based on this external exam. This happens all the time. The folks in the ER don't realize we can't do that right after childbirth."

Wait. We tell women to go to the ER if they have concerning symptoms, but if they do, it's pretty much common knowledge that the providers there don't know much about childbirth? Is this why maternal mortality is so high in the U.S.?

We finished the ultrasound, and I was wheeled back to our small, dreary, windowless room (only notable because, *the day before*, I'd been discharged from the Ritz-Carlton-esque birth center of the very same hospital). I couldn't help but feel that the stark difference in environment reflected a difference in my value, as well as in the care I was likely to receive.

After five hours of my husband and I trading off holding Julian, I started to feel myself getting sleepy. I envisioned, with horror, one of us falling asleep while holding him and dropping him on the hard floor.

I wished there were somewhere we could put Julian down safely, but the room contained only the tall, side-less hospital bed, some medical supplies, an extra chair, and our car seat.

Before you ask… No, the car seat didn't feel like an option to me at the time. Why? Because it's drilled in *hard* to new parents that the car seat is not a safe place to leave your baby unless you're actually in the car.

It was 1 a.m., and I was sobbing.

I went out to the hallways to plead with whoever would listen for somewhere safe where I could put my baby down.

The response I got was, "Hmm… We don't have that kind of thing in the ER. We don't see a lot of babies."

What do you mean, you don't see a lot of babies? Am I the first postpartum mom who has ever come here while still (essentially) physically attached to their baby?

A short while later, a kind young woman came rushing in with a baby scale outfitted with a few blankets in an attempt at a makeshift bassinet.

She was doing her best to come up with a solution to my problem, and I respect that. My problem here is with "my people": hospital administration. Why did this woman need to jerry-rig a janky bassinet for my baby? I gave birth at a Level I trauma center in a major metro area in one of the wealthiest countries in the world. Why wasn't it easier to obtain a bassinet for a new mother holding a days-old baby?

All ERs in the United States should be outfitted with basic postpartum supplies. This way, when we tell new moms that they should come in for "maternal danger signs X, Y, and Z," we actually mean it, regardless of whether they're privileged enough to have family available who make it possible for them to leave their baby at home.

We've got a lot of expensive, hard-to-solve problems in healthcare. This is not one of them.

Eventually, what felt like hours later, someone came in and told us I was okay to leave, and that they were going to prescribe me a few medications. One to help stop the bleeding, and one to help reduce my blood pressure.

Now, I'd been watching my blood pressure at home like a *hawk* throughout my pregnancy, given my fear of dying in childbirth and my elevated risk of pre-eclampsia due to family history. Fortunately, despite my concerns, it had never been an issue.

"No," I responded to the ER provider at my door. "My blood pressure is probably high because this has been an extremely stressful experience and I'm terrified for both myself and my baby. I don't want to be discharged until we see someone from OB."

I was emphatic, and I'd temporarily put aside my typical filter.

You have made it abundantly clear that you know nothing about childbirth. I do not want to leave without knowing that someone who's familiar with the process of childbirth tells me it's safe for me to do so. There are way too many stories of pregnant or postpartum women being sent home from the ER only to die a few hours later. I will not be one of them.[v]

Eventually, in the wee hours of the morning, the OB team came in to evaluate me and review my records.

I tearfully explained how the night had gone and why I was so anxious. They told me that they were sorry, and that they knew that coming to the ER is far from ideal for newly postpartum moms. They confirmed that I was safe to leave and agreed that we could hold the blood pressure medication until we had a chance to re-test in the morning (with the at-home blood pressure machine I had due to the aforementioned blood pressure fears).

---

[v]   Keep this in mind when I reach the point of suicidal ideation just a week or so later. At this juncture, I was frantically self-advocating in an attempt to continue living.

CHAPTER 3

The Descent

My anxiety over the smallest of tasks, which began in the hospital with the car seat instructions, continued to grow throughout our first week at home.

From the start, I didn't want to be the one to clean the breast pump or bottle parts.

If I don't do this right, Julian could get a nasty infection and die. It would be my fault. I'm definitely not doing this right. Somebody else who's more competent should do this.

Each time Julian was in his car seat, I would worry about his airway closing. As discussed previously, you aren't supposed to let babies sleep in their car seat unless they're in the car.[15]

But what's so different about the car seat being in the car, really? Maybe the truth is that the risk is always there, but they don't say that because we live in America and they know people have to drive. So, instead, they just say to only use the car seat if you're driving. It would probably be best to watch Julian whenever we're driving in the car, so I can intervene if he spontaneously stops breathing...

Most of all, I worried about him sleeping. I never wanted to be the last one to touch him before he went to sleep.

If I swaddle him too tightly or too loosely, he could die of sudden infant death syndrome (SIDS). I can't risk that. I should get someone else to swaddle him, or at the very least to double- and triple-check my work each time.

I started to have trouble sleeping at night because I didn't like all of us to be asleep at once.

What if he stops breathing and neither of us notices? I can't let that happen. This baby is now my everything. I wouldn't be able to live with that amount of sadness. I'll just watch him until Alex wakes up or my mom comes over.

Over time, this anxiety started to pour over my brain and take on a life of its own, seemingly untethered to any specific worry or concern. It was with me all day, and eventually it was with me all night, too. I would go to sleep at night only to wake up an hour or two later, teeming with anxiety I couldn't shake, despite not having slept through the night in several weeks.

"I Get It Now"

By one week postpartum, I knew something was very wrong. I was vacillating between two states of being: one semi-"normal," and one marked by panic and hopelessness. The "normal" me began desperately trying to fight back.

Below is a note from my phone that "normal me" wrote to "panic me," the latter of which was sure that I didn't have interests or hobbies or things to do to pass the time between feedings:

June 2023 (Julian is 8 days old)

Things to do

Laundry

Find something decorative on Etsy for Julian's room

Bake bread, zucchini bread, cookies, etc.

Work on a baby book or scrapbook for Julian

Play Sporcle to brush up on countries/capitals/bodies
of water/etc.

Read a book for fun

Read a book about parenting

Learn how to cook something

Look through yearbooks

Snuggle with Howie

Call someone

Watch a new show on Netflix

Work on my Spanish

Journal my thoughts/experiences

Work on something for Alex for Father's Day

Upper body exercises

Take a shower

Listen to a podcast

Get some sun on the porch

I remember telling Alex during a "normal" moment, "I'm not suicidal, but now I understand it. I've never understood how someone could make that choice, but now I do."

I thought I was being honest, because in the moment when I shared that with him, I wasn't feeling suicidal. But in retrospect, those thoughts had been starting to come in my hardest moments, which is why I now understood.

If you're someone who can't quite comprehend how and why people die by suicide, I understand, because that was me for the first 27 years of my life. I don't think that you're a bad person, and I don't think that you lack compassion. Just please try to take my word for it that your incomprehension is a gift: one that reflects the fact that you haven't personally experienced the lowest of lows that depression and anxiety have to offer.

***

Fear wasn't the only thing causing my distress. I also found myself unbearably overwhelmed by Julian's cries and the never-ending loop of menial tasks that were now required of me.

I frequently found myself wanting to escape, and I was terrified at the realization that I couldn't just quietly disappear for a few hours of alone time whenever I found myself overwhelmed and overstimulated to the point of functional paralysis.[vi] I hadn't realized that this had been one of my regular coping tools until the moment when it became inaccessible.

And, of course, along with this desire to escape the noise, the cries, and the mundane tasks came the guilt associated with that feeling.

A good mom would not feel this way. A good mom would not be overwhelmed by her baby's cries. A good mom would not resent having to do all of the newborn tasks.

My mom spent a lot of time with us in that first week, which I'm extremely grateful for. I know many people don't have support like that. And (because my therapist has given

---

vi   Yes, to anyone who raised an eyebrow here, I've come to realize that I probably have some degree of attention deficit hyperactivity disorder (ADHD), which nobody ever suspected because I excelled in school and didn't act out very often as a child.

me permission to feel multiple, sometimes conflicting, things at once) having my mom around all the time was also challenging. Not because I didn't want and need her help, but because in the absence of a clear, healthy perspective, her presence became fuel for comparison and harsh self-judgment.

My mom doesn't seem overwhelmed by my baby's cries. My mom seems like she'd be happy to change diapers and feed babies all day long. Maybe she should just take care of him. He deserves a mom like her, not a selfish, lazy mom like me.

Hindsight note: Here's the perspective I was missing at the time: I was a first-time mom, with zero infant experience, recovering from childbirth, severe blood loss, and prolonged sleep deprivation. My mom, on the other hand, had raised four children, had not just endured a major medical event, and was eating, drinking, and sleeping as usual. It wasn't even remotely a fair comparison for me to be making. But alas.

Losing My Ability to Eat

My appetite had slowly been disappearing since we arrived home. I was relying on meal replacement drinks to sustain me, because not only was I not hungry, but my body was starting to become unwilling and unable to consume food.

I'd struggled with disordered eating in my past, so this brought up a whole new crop of concerns.

Is it coming back? Am I developing an eating disorder? Was I completely wrong in my previous understanding of eating disorders: real eating disorders are actually when you just physically stop being able to take in nutrition?

> **Hindsight note:** No. But losing your appetite *is* an incredibly common symptom of postpartum anxiety.[16]

I would try to force down a meal, knowing full well that my body needed nutrition, only to throw it all up shortly afterward.

Ice cream was one of the only things I was able to eat and keep down, which reminded me of my grandmother in the final days and weeks of her life while battling Alzheimer's.

My body is literally shutting down. This is a sign that I'm dying.

When I was awake, despite the fact that I wasn't keeping much food or water down anymore, I felt like I had to constantly be moving or doing something. So, we took a lot of walks: sometimes up to four or five miles a day, according to my Apple Health records.

One morning, I tried to take some hydroxyzine (the only tool I'd been offered thus far by medical providers to help manage my acute anxiety) with water. But immediately after I swallowed, I ran toward the bathroom, though I didn't quite make it. I threw up all of the water, including the pills, which were still fully intact.

My husband, also lost and confused about what was going on, was frustrated by this. So, he offered up one of the least useful statements imaginable: "You need to keep that down."[vii]

It's too late. Nothing can help me now.

---

vii   Yes, I've since teased him about this plenty. He has been generous in allowing me to share his less-than-ideal moments in this book, too.

Scary Thoughts

Around the time all of this was happening, my brain had started bombarding me with scary thoughts and images of death and dying. At one point, I told my husband, "My brain is giving me pictures of you as a single dad."

I didn't want to be alone. I knew I wasn't in control of my thoughts, and I figured it was only a matter of time before I wouldn't be in control of my actions, either.

I've read the headlines. I'm turning into some sort of crazy person. Is this psychosis? What if I wake up one day and want to kill my husband?

Cue abhorrent mental images of me murdering my family, whom I love more than anything in the world, and then intense fear and horror about that (supposed) possibility.

Hindsight note: While this book is mostly a critique of the healthcare industry and its leaders, I also have some strong feelings about journalists. Please stop publishing the gruesome postpartum psychosis clickbait that's actually a reflection of tragic illnesses that we've failed to screen for and adequately treat, rather than of monsters among us. When you publish these articles, you're revealing your own ignorance of the topic and making it harder for people to speak up and get help when they're struggling.

Seeking Help

You might think that because I work in healthcare administration, and because my husband is a physician, we'd have known exactly what was happening and what we should do.

That was, unfortunately, not the case in the slightest.

I was furiously Googling "postpartum depression" but struggling to find validation that the things I was experiencing—the inability to eat or drink, for example—was a symptom of that. And I *wasn't* experiencing some of the "classic" symptoms, like crying all day or feeling deep sadness, so we didn't recognize what was going on.

As a healthcare administrator, I heard all the time about how difficult it is to access behavioral health and how it can take months. I knew in my heart that I didn't have months to wait, so I had my husband call the Behavioral Health scheduling line of the health system where I worked, received my regular OB care, and delivered my baby (which I'll call Large Nonprofit Health System) on my behalf.

He did, and sure enough, he was told it would be a few months before I could be seen. He asked whether there were any exceptions for OB patients and was told no. He hung up without making an appointment, because we both knew that waiting months was out of the question.

I went into the clinic for a mood check about 10 days after getting home from the hospital. The visit was with a doctor I'd never seen before, because in American healthcare, access is awful; it's nearly impossible to see who you want to see when you want to see them.[viii]

I was weighed, and I was down nearly 30 pounds (nearly 20% of my body weight) from when I'd delivered my baby a week and a half before.

Nobody said anything about that.

---

viii   I recognize that the same is true of other countries; we just do it at twice the cost while *claiming* that we reap the benefits of free market efficiency.

That visit was the first time I had a "positive screen" on the Edinburgh Postnatal Depression Scale (EPDS), a standardized questionnaire used to detect postpartum depression. In disbelief and overcome with shame, I answered honestly the final question about whether I was having thoughts of self-harm: "yes."

Checking that box was one of the scariest, most vulnerable things I've ever done.

I had no history of clinical mental illness. Checking the box was an unavoidable reminder that something foreign had taken over me. It was something I knew I could never take back, that would be in my medical history forever. I didn't know what, if any, implications there were in checking that box.

What do they do with women who are such terrible humans that becoming a mother makes them think about killing themselves?[ix]

I just knew I needed, and desperately wanted, help.

The nursing assistant who first saw my responses to the form was kind: she looked me in the eye, softened her voice, and thanked me for being honest.

But the doctor who came in a few minutes later was different. She was nonchalant about the EPDS results, simply noting that she'd placed an urgent behavioral health referral for me and that they would follow up.

She seemed fixated on the fact that I'd elected not to take the blood pressure medication that had been prescribed to me

---

ix   Please remember that this is a distorted thought. Thoughts of self-harm do not make you a terrible human, no matter the circumstance. The correct answer to this question *should* be, "give them compassionate, evidence-based care."

in the ER a few days earlier,[x] and she was far more concerned about that than about my mood symptoms. She also told me that the health system had a 24/7 crisis line that I could use if needed, which would connect me in real time with a counselor.

I walked out of that appointment even more anxious than when I'd walked in. I'd taken what felt like an enormous step—disclosing that I was having thoughts of self-harm—and, essentially, nothing had happened. The doctor didn't seem to think much of it, and clearly felt that giving me a referral and sending on my way was an appropriate response.

So, I just walked out the door, alone and terrified of what the future held.

The *next* day, I got a call from the behavioral health department, as promised. I was offered an appointment on Monday, which was six days away.

They must not understand. I can't eat, I can't sleep, I have uncontrollable diarrhea, and I'm having scary thoughts all day long. I don't have six days in me, and even if I did, there's no chance that a one-hour conversation with someone can fix whatever's going on with me.

The next day, I sent a message to my normal OB provider, the one I'd seen at least 10 times throughout my pregnancy. "I'm not doing very well… I have no appetite, and I threw up today after trying to force myself to eat lunch," I wrote. To which I received a message from a nurse that said, "I checked with Behavioral Health to see if they had any sooner therapy appointments for you, and they currently do not."

---

x   Despite my blood pressure returning to normal the morning after I was discharged from the ER, as anticipated.

Hindsight note: Why didn't this person suggest that I seek care outside of the system? I now know that Postpartum Support International (PSI) has a free online directory of certified perinatal mental health providers. And where I live, the chances are high that one of them would've had rapid availability, and undoubtedly sooner than six days. This experience has opened my eyes to the dark side of the "come here and get all of your care under one roof" obsession that has gripped U.S. healthcare leaders, including and *especially* the Large Nonprofit Health System leaders, over the last decade or so.

This same day, I also had my second lactation appointment, because despite everything I was experiencing, I was still trying my hardest to breastfeed my son. During this appointment, I shared with the lactation consultant that I was having trouble eating and drinking, and I asked if that was going to have an impact on my ability to breastfeed.

In retrospect, this was a cry for help more than it was a genuine question. I was trying to find a way to alert someone about the scary symptoms I was having, without having to directly admit once again that I was struggling and really needed help.

"Don't worry; your baby will be just fine," she told me. "They've actually done studies on starving women in Africa and found that even women who are physically starving can breastfeed their children successfully," she continued.

"Okay," I nodded weakly, aware even in my half-functioning state that her response was extraordinarily odd and inappropriate on multiple levels.

After that appointment, I broke down in the car. The lactation consultant had told us to prepare for a growth spurt. I said to my husband, "He's growing so fast, and I'm missing all of it."

"What do you mean? You're not missing it; you're right here," my husband said, trying to comfort me.

But I wasn't. I wasn't myself, and I'd lost my ability to feel joy. I was missing all of it.

Hanging On by a Thread

Later that day, I received a call from a concerned nurse at my OB's office who told me that she, too, had been to a dark place after the birth of one of her children. She pleaded with me to stay safe and get help.

That call was important to me. It was one of the few times I felt seen in my suffering. But it still didn't help me understand what "help" she, or anyone else, was referencing. I'd been to the clinic multiple times, and I was trying unsuccessfully to get into therapy. None of it was helping.

Maybe I've called their bluff, and they don't actually know how to help people with this.

Despite these feelings and fears, I continued frantically trying to convince myself that I was okay, hoping that I could calm myself down.

If you need proof, here's another relic from my Notes app:

June 2023 (Julian is 13 days old)
Things have gotten better.
I no longer have nausea.
I no longer have pubic symphysis pain.
I no longer have to fear birth.
I no longer have heartburn.
I can see again, I can walk again.

It no longer stings to pee.
It no longer hurts to sit straight down.
I can breastfeed successfully now.
I can change diapers now.
I can confidently handle/hold Julian's head now.
I am less anxious about Julian breathing while sleeping than I was before.
I am less anxious about other health issues related to Julian than I was before.
I have taken care of insurance needs.

Hindsight note: My heart aches for this version of myself. She was fighting this battle so, so hard. Now, whenever I hear about a woman who's passed away after a battle with postpartum depression or anxiety, I think about how hard she was probably trying to hang on. It is devastating beyond words.

That night, as had become the norm, I had trouble sleeping. I got out of bed and tried calling the 24/7 crisis line whose details I'd been given multiple times.

"You have reached the Behavioral Health appointment scheduling line. Our business hours are from 8 a.m. to 5 p.m., Monday through Friday. If this is an emergency, please call 911."

I took this as additional evidence that whatever I was suffering from was unknown and rare.

If this was a real thing, the doctors wouldn't be handing out the number of a nonexistent crisis line. Somebody would have said something. I must be the first one.

The day after that, things were getting worse, and my thoughts were continuing to get darker. At one point, I said to my husband while writhing on the couch, "I think there's only one way this ends. Maybe I should do it soon so that you can start moving on with your life more quickly."

By this point, I felt like I was living in a tragic movie whose ending I already knew. I felt certain that I was going to die; I just didn't know how yet. I was consumed with anticipatory grief for my family and with extraordinary guilt for the role I thought I was playing in that grief.

Julian's life will be defined by the trauma of losing his mom so early, to suicide no less. I can't believe I'm doing that to him. It's my fault that I'm not strong enough to survive this. How many days of frozen breastmilk do we have? I wish I had more to leave him.

My mom was deeply concerned at this point and helped me make yet another OB appointment, this time with her at my side. I saw another new OB provider, because, again, access is terrible, which is the rule and not the exception.

At this appointment, I was offered the EPDS again, and this time I refused. I knew that responding to the questions was only going to heighten my fears about what was happening to me and what I thought the inevitable outcome was going to be.

I remember telling that doctor, "I feel like I'm fighting to survive 22 hours a day." The only thing she offered was to refill the hydroxyzine that I'd started while in the hospital and to tell me that I should go to the ER "if I felt I was truly in danger."

What could they possibly do for me at the ER? They'll put me in a "safe" room where I can't hurt myself, but there's no way they have any tools that could help me actually feel better. If they did, someone would've thought to mention that to me by now.

Given my previous experience with the ER following the blood clot, the concept that they would know what was happening to me and how to help was completely implausible to me.

As I described to my husband, by this point, what I was experiencing was "like the worst physical pain I've ever experienced, but in my head." I pictured the ER and the hospital as just a way to force me to continue living in agony but without the ability to escape it in the only way I could currently imagine, which was death.

"Can you ask them to put me into a coma while they try to figure out what to do?" I asked my husband, knowing the answer was "no" but figuring it was worth a shot.

Again, we went home, with nothing but a vague promise of resources to be provided later via MyChart.

Nobody knows what to do with me. The only possible explanation is that they've never seen this before, or at least they've never seen anyone recover from this before. They must know that there's nothing they can offer to help me.

On the way home from that appointment, my mom and I stopped at Target. It was early June. Father's Day was coming up, and so was my wedding anniversary. It dawned on me that instead of celebrating either of those occasions together, my husband would be spending them alone, caring for a newborn all by himself, drowning in grief.

Would it make it better or worse if I left him a card?

It was later that evening that I reached the lowest point of my journey.

CHAPTER 4

The Bottom

That night, as usual, I woke up soon after falling asleep. The pain in my head (I have no better words for it, though it was quite different from a headache) was unbearable. I considered waking my husband, but I knew he needed sleep to care for our baby, and I knew he was as confused and lost as I was about what was happening to me.

I got out of bed, hugged my dog, and went to the nursery.

I sat in the rocking chair, scrolling my phone, desperately searching for evidence that anyone had ever recovered from something like what I was feeling and experiencing. Plenty of articles came up with similarities to my story.

Yes, this sounds like me… yes… yes…

But many, if not most, of them ended in tragedy.

I'll spare you the details, but to this day, I remember what happened to the women in the articles I read that night.

And I remember the overwhelming panic, guilt, and dread as I concluded—definitively—that this must be how my story would end, too.

So that night, I began the *devastating* process of thinking about my options for ending my life and trying to figure out which one would minimize the pain for everyone involved.

I hope you never find yourself in that place.

No amount of therapy, medication, or time will change the fact that I've now been to that particular dark corner in my mind. The only silver lining to that experience being a part of my memory and my life story is that I now have a completely different level of compassion for others who've been there too, as well as the fire in my heart to fight for them.

Later that night, Alex found me in the fetal position on the ground in the nursery, having just gotten off the phone with the suicide hotline. He had woken up, realized that my side of the bed was empty, and come looking for me.

He's a physician, and at the time, he was beginning his final year of medical school. He's also just a good Samaritan. He knew the basics of what he needed to say and do.

He asked me if I was thinking of suicide, and I nodded.

He asked if I had a plan, and I said, "No, but I am thinking about it. I'm so scared. I don't want it to hurt. It already hurts so much."

He knew that I didn't want to go to the ER, because we'd discussed this option after the latest doctor's appointment. I explained, tearfully, that I desperately wanted help, but I didn't want to go to the ER because I knew that wasn't the answer. And I knew I wouldn't be able to bring my baby. Holding my baby was one of the only effective tools I had for reducing my anxiety, even if just the tiniest amount.

By that point, Alex had worked in several different ERs as a scribe, a technician, and a medical student. He knew that there was some truth to my fears.

He asked me to take some of an old Ativan prescription we had in the house for my flying phobia to help me get to sleep and get through the night. I did, and with the help of the medication, I was able to get a few consecutive hours of sleep, which was the most I'd had in at least 24 hours.

As soon as I fell asleep, Alex called my mom and shared what had happened. She came over immediately, so that there would always be one person responsible for Julian and one person responsible for me.

In the morning, my mom called my aunt, a nurse who lives in another state. She shared what was going on, how I'd been acting, and what I'd been saying. My aunt calmly and clearly stated that I needed to go to the ER. She asked to talk to me.

She told me she knew I was hurting. She told me she knew I was scared. She told me that this was something that could happen to new moms, and that we would find someone who could help me, even if we hadn't been able to find that person yet. And she told me that what I needed to do, for myself and for my family, was go to the ER.

Sobbing, I hung up the phone and found my husband. "I need to go to the ER," I told him. He nodded, and we started packing up a bag.

How many pairs of clothes do I need? How do you pack for this? Can I bring my razor? Why do I care about shaving my legs if I'm also thinking about killing myself? This is so confusing.

I was torn between hope and despair, not knowing whether I would be there one night or forever.

The hardest part was kissing my tiny, two-week-old baby goodbye, and telling him that I loved him so, so, so much. I left not knowing when I would get to see him again.

My Inpatient Stay on a General Psychiatric Unit

Checking into the ER was, surprisingly, one of the few bright spots in my early journey. The woman at the desk asked what I was there for, and softly, I said, "I'm here for suicidal ideation. I just had a baby two weeks ago," with my head hanging low.

The woman looked me directly in the eyes and said, "Thank you for coming here. Thank you for getting help."

I started sobbing all over again.

I sat in the waiting room with my husband. It was about noon on a Friday. The waiting room scared me, so I put my metaphorical blinders on and tried not to look around.

Fortunately, we were called back fairly quickly (a rare gift from the universe, I know). After a brief triage, they brought me to another section of the unit and asked me to place my belongings in a locker. They told me that was where my husband would wait, and that I needed to go to the back with them alone.

Cue more tears.

I was placed in a room and told that someone would be in shortly.

I was alone with my thoughts: the scariest place I could imagine. Eventually, after I talked with a few people, my husband was allowed in the room with me. We were given some puzzles and something to write with. I lay on the twin bed with my husband, working on a sudoku puzzle. I felt deeply ashamed.

How can I be casually working on a puzzle with my favorite person in the world while also having racing thoughts about death and hurting myself?

I felt like a traitor to my husband, who is without question the most supportive, loving spouse I could have ever asked for (in spite of that one unhelpful comment regarding throwing up my anxiety meds).

At some point, a staff member walked by my room and glanced at me. She stopped in her tracks, got a smile on her face, and said, "Hi! It's good to see you again!"

I stared at her, not knowing what to say.

"Remember me, from last time?" she continued.

"No, I've never been here before," I responded through more tears.

As was now the norm, the spiral came quickly.

Is this life for me now: bouncing between home and the psychiatric unit of the ER? Even if I manage to get discharged, am I bound to come right back?

That thought was devastating.

Ultimately, I was admitted voluntarily to an inpatient psychiatric unit. I was promised that it was family-friendly and that my family, including my son, could come visit me each day.

The reason I opted so easily for admission was less about me and more about reducing the perceived burden on my family. I felt *enormously* guilty for the stress my situation was causing my family, and I figured that being admitted would remove some of that, at least temporarily.

We went up to the unit, and they showed me my room. They explained some of the rules: no devices, no shoelaces, no razors. Someone would check on me every 15 minutes, day and night.

Again, the spirals came quickly.

I had a breast pump with me, which had a charger cord. Nobody said anything about it or took it away from me.

I'm not supposed to have this. That must be because if I have this, I might develop an urge to hurt myself with it.

I made my husband take the cord home with him.

Let that sink in: I was admitted to an inpatient psychiatric unit for active suicidal ideation, yet I told my husband to take the breast pump cord home with him because I was so scared of hurting myself with it.

I assume this is why people often say that suicidal ideation comes from an urge to escape desperate pain, not from a desire to die. I can't speak for others, and I'm not an expert on this subject by any means, but I can speak for myself: this was 100% true for me.

There were moments, more than I'd like to admit, during my journey with postpartum anxiety and depression when I thought about ending my life. And if that option had been easier to access, I really might have done it.

But it was never—not once—because I *wanted* that to be the outcome. It was because I didn't believe that the pain I was feeling would ever end, and I knew that I couldn't bear to withstand it forever. In those moments, death felt like the only humane option.

Each night, I was separated from Julian and my family.

I remember the first night like it was yesterday. My husband stayed until the last possible moment, and then the staff started reminding us that visiting hours were over. He said goodnight, and then he and Julian headed home without me.

You know that feeling when you feel so much sadness that the lump in your throat genuinely hurts and almost makes you feel like you're suffocating?

That was how I felt that first night.

A very kind nurse walked the halls with me as I cried and tried to regain my composure.

That night, I woke up to pump, and I brought my breastmilk in a labeled bag to the desk for refrigeration. It took a little bit of time for me to get anyone to look me in the eye. It was the most dehumanizing experience I've ever had in my life, and it's one that I now think about every time I pass an unhoused person on the street and have the urge to avert my eyes.

But once I did catch someone's attention, they seemed confused. "Breastmilk? To refrigerate?"

"Please, just take it to the back," I said. "I've been handing it in all day. I know there's a refrigerator back there."

Experiences like this on the inpatient unit, just like my experiences in the clinic, gave me the impression that I was the first to ever walk this road.

In addition to some staff members raising an eyebrow in response to being handed breastmilk, some seemed scandalized by walking in on me pumping or breastfeeding—something that happened often, given the frequency of the wellness checks and the frequency with which newborns eat.

One of the very few times I cracked a smile during the first month of Julian's life was on a day when my mom was visiting me at the hospital. I was sharing with her how unfamiliar and uncomfortable some of the staff members, particularly men, seemed regarding breastfeeding and handling breast milk.

"Just imagine if I went up to one of them in the middle of the night and asked them if they could please go get me some nipple cream," I said. We both laughed.

———

I struggle to write about my time in the inpatient unit, because I want to avoid further stigmatization. So first, let me be clear: individuals in psychiatric units are sick, just like patients with cancer are sick, and they deserve care and respect. Nobody, and I mean nobody, would elect to have a mental health disorder: it's a disease, and a cruel one at that.

But in my opinion, it's also true that being thrust into a general inpatient psychiatric unit is a horrible way to be introduced to the world of mental health disorders and mental healthcare. It doesn't set you up for maximum compassion and understanding; it sets you up for fear and othering.

As established, at this point in my life, the spirals came quickly, and they came often.

I remember looking out of the tiny window in my room, feeling like Princess Fiona locked up in the Highest Room of the Tallest Tower.

What if I never feel sunlight again?

For most of my time on the unit, I stayed hidden away in my little room. One morning, I worked up the courage to go to the communal breakfast room. An older woman, in hospital-issued clothing, missing a few teeth, and slightly disheveled, said to me, "I know this place sucks. But the good thing about being here is that we're the only ones who understand each other."

I was crushed.

Tears filled my eyes immediately.

No, I don't understand you. And you don't understand me.

Three weeks ago, I was unpacking my new home, preparing for my new baby, touring hospitals like this one in business clothes, and going out to eat with my husband. Then childbirth broke me. But I do not belong here.

… or do I?

Is this the secret behind the world of mental illness? People just wake up one day and cease to have the ability to function? And nobody knows what to do about it or how to help them, so we just lock them up in a unit and take away their means to an end? Maybe I am "one of them" now. Maybe I'll be "one of them" for the rest of my life, if I keep living.

I hope that kind woman got the care she needed and is doing better now. I'm embarrassed about how I reacted when she tried to relate to me, but I'm sharing it anyway because my intention with this book is to be radically transparent, even about the moments that make me hurt or cringe in hindsight. Fear has a way of bringing out the worst in people.

These are simply the real, unfiltered thoughts that I had while trying to make sense of my new reality. As you can see, the spirals came quickly and often, and they went very, very deep.

My inpatient stay was traumatizing in itself; there's no doubt about that. But given the circumstances I was in at the time, I'm thankful that I went to the ER and that I accepted the recommendation of admission. Being hospitalized helped keep me safe while I was in crisis, and it bought my family time to do some research into treatment options.

It was during this time that my mom found out that there was actually a partial hospitalization program (PHP) designed specifically for pregnant and postpartum women only 15 minutes from home at a competitor health system that I'll call Other Local Health System.

You might think that this news instantly dampened my fears and helped me feel confident that I would recover, but that wasn't the case. By this point, I was *so certain* that the concept of "help" was a farce that I found it impossible to believe that this perinatal PHP would be effective.

It didn't matter that the woman my mom spoke to on the phone claimed that they saw women like me all the time, or that they said they had confidence they could help me. All I knew was that people kept promising hope, telling me to just hold on, and then offering me absolutely nothing. It was going to take a lot of convincing to get me to believe otherwise.

But that said, I was willing to try the program.

As I explained to my mom one day while she was visiting—likely to her horror—I didn't believe it would work, but I was willing to try it, because my family deserved for me to try any and all options before ending my life. The enormous amount of guilt that I felt about the impending tragedy I believed I was leaving my family with was assuaged ever so slightly by this concept.

I'm not going to survive this. But this program gives me another thing to try, another way to show my family that I love them and am willing to try anything to stay with them. I owe that to them.

CHAPTER 5

The Climb

Perinatal Partial Hospitalization Program

Fortunately, I was completely and entirely wrong in thinking that nobody could help me.

In retrospect, the concept of help only felt like a farce because I hadn't actually been offered any help yet.

It is not an exaggeration to say that the moment we found the perinatal partial hospitalization program (PHP), my entire trajectory changed.

The program I attended offered programming for five hours a day, four days a week. It was group therapy based and included psychotherapy, psychoeducation, trauma-informed yoga classes, parenting education, and parenting support. Each patient also had an individual therapist they saw weekly, as well as the opportunity to see a perinatal psychiatrist several days each week.

The most incredible and unique aspect of the PHP, for me, was the ability to bring your baby. Bringing your baby wasn't just allowed; it was encouraged and actively supported. The program was equipped with nursing supplies, baby toys, bassinets, and helping hands. The staff empowered me to care for my baby, and they were also prepared to offer caregiving assistance at any time.

The earliest that they could get me into the program was in two weeks, but they arranged for me to come in to complete the intake paperwork and create a safety plan the day after I was discharged from the inpatient unit.

That first day was both wonderful and deeply disappointing. I came in with my family, filled out all of the obligatory paperwork and screening forms (a very sensitive exercise for me), and then spent the better part of an hour talking through everything that had happened and creating a safety plan with a therapist.

But then that was it: our session was over, and it was time to go home.

I remember panicking and telling the extremely kind therapist, "I don't feel any better; I'm actually feeling much worse," to which she responded, "Oh, I'm so sorry. I should have explained at the beginning. This is just an intake; this isn't really the therapeutic part."

So, my intake day was wonderful, because it was my first time feeling seen, validated, and truly cared for—but it was also disappointing, because the concept of actually feeling any better as the result of an interaction with professionals still eluded me. It turns out intake appointments can be pretty rough.[xi]

A few days later, I had my first individual perinatal psychiatry visit with the psychiatrist who'd founded the program a decade prior, whom I'll call Dr. E.

I'll never forget that first visit. Dr. E was the very first medical professional out of the dozens I'd seen to date on my journey to tell me that she[xii] knew exactly what was happening

---

xi   This is feedback that I've still never given to Other Local Health System, because I'm now wary of healthcare leaders and organizations turning their back on me the moment I offer feedback of the constructive, rather than pat-on-the-back, variety.

xii   I originally used gender-neutral pronouns for all of the healthcare leaders in this book. But then I checked the online Postpartum Support International (PSI) provider directory and found that only five out of the hundreds of perinatal psychiatrists they have listed are men. So, I've decided there's no need to dance around the fact that the leader of this PHP was a woman.

to me, and that she had confidence that she could help guide me to recovery. She also told me that she had tools to help me right away, not just in several months, as I'd been told before.

I wanted more than anything in the world to believe what she was telling me: that she knew what was going on with me and could help me recover. But I was highly skeptical.

If you know how much I'm suffering, and if this is as common as you're telling me it is, then why did so many people along this journey look at me and shrug their shoulders? It can't be true. There's no way. Our healthcare system has problems, but it's not THAT bad.

I also held a lot of (common) misconceptions about what postpartum depression was and who could get it.

Yes, I've heard of postpartum depression. But aren't the risk factors for postpartum depression things like minimal social support and history of mental illness? Those don't apply to me. I don't have that. I'm too privileged to have postpartum depression. I'm just a horrible mom.

I struggled to believe that what I was experiencing was postpartum depression. I thought I didn't have the "right" to claim a label like that—one that assigns the blame to an illness. I thought that while *some* women were legitimately sick, I wasn't; I was simply not cut out for motherhood. And that in my case, calling it postpartum depression would be making excuses for a problem that was actually just a sign of my selfishness and other character flaws.

Another thing I struggled with in the early days of the PHP was my interpretation of the concept that my thinking patterns may have been causing my distress. I took this as an indication that I was personally responsible for the enormous distress I was feeling.

After all, we choose our thoughts, right?

Hindsight note: No, we do not choose all of our thoughts. It would have been nice to learn that a bit earlier in my life.

As established, I'd never been to therapy before. I also come from a high-achieving family, where, growing up, I learned both implicitly and explicitly that I'm a "good" critical thinker—and, therefore, that the conclusions I draw when I've thought long and hard about something are, more often than not, correct.

The concept that my thoughts, such as my extensively thought-out and rationalized conclusion that I was suffering from a rare and unknown condition that had no cure, were perhaps "untrue" didn't seem plausible.

I'm not an idiot. The doctors don't know what to do with me. If doctor after doctor after doctor doesn't know what to do with me, this must not be common or curable. Besides, even if this was related to my mental health, a switch flipped when my baby was born. My body is literally shutting down. I can't eat or sleep, and I have uncontrollable diarrhea.[xiii] It's not all in my head.

---

xiii   Remember that scene in *Bridesmaids* where the bride has food poisoning and starts pooping in the middle of the street, saying, "It's happening! It's happening!"? That was me as a new mom. Whether it was the anxiety or a side effect of the SSRI I had started the day Julian was born, I'll never know.

Eventually, after repeated suggestions that perhaps I *did* have some underlying mental health issues, primarily related to anxiety, I started panic-accepting this reality.

Okay, fine; maybe I am messed up. Once this is all over (if it's ever all over), I'll get help. I'll go to therapy. I promise. But for now, I just want to go back to how I was pre-delivery, even if it's not perfect. I just want to go back to the version of me that could eat and sleep, and that had bowel continence.

It took me a long time to comprehend the fact that several seemingly conflicting things can be true at once. One of which is that you can be an extremely intelligent, excellent critical thinker and *also* have your thinking clouded by mental health disorders like anxiety and depression.

It also took me a long time to comprehend (as you'll see in Part 2) the fact that just because a condition is common doesn't mean that the American healthcare system is prepared to address it.

The fact that none of the doctors I interacted with during my two-week high-speed downward spiral knew what to do with me was not a reflection of the rarity and poor prognosis of my condition; rather, it was a reflection of the fact that both women's health and mental health are undervalued and under-resourced in the U.S. healthcare system.

And the intersection of both—well, that's even worse.

On my first day of the group therapy program, I was terrified. Since I'd never been to therapy before, let alone group therapy, I had no idea what to say or what to expect.

I walked in and saw a woman smiling and caring competently for her older infant, who clearly loved his mom and saw her as a beacon of safety and happiness.

Why is she here? She seems like she's doing so well. She seems like a much more confident and capable parent than me.

Hindsight note: This woman has become one of my good friends, so I know now that she was decidedly *not* doing so well at that particular moment in her life. Looks can be deceiving, and you never know what battles someone is fighting internally.

I don't remember much from that first day, but I know that I was reserved, and that I held everything and everyone at arm's length.

A few days in, I remember my voice starting to quiver as I spoke about something.

Another woman, who's also now a close friend, said, "Emily, it's okay to cry. You're safe to cry here. Everything about this sucks. Let it out."

I started sobbing.

Looking back, one of the most amazing transformations of my maternal mental health recovery journey was that it taught me how to actually feel my emotions, and to let go—mostly, anyway—of my concerns about what others will think if I *show* that I do, in fact, have emotions.

I hate to admit it, but I harbored some pretty deep judgments about the other moms when I first started the program.

I remember one young single mom mentioning that she co-slept with her child. Another young single mom saw that as an opportunity to share that she, too, co-slept with her baby.

OMG, is somebody going to say something? Haven't they heard that co-sleeping is incredibly dangerous? If they're as anxious as they claim to be, how on Earth are they choosing to co-sleep?

Yikes. Who was I—a mom with a safe and available co-parent and a strong support system, who was also actively feeling the repercussions of significant and prolonged sleep deprivation—to judge a young single mom for doing what she needed to survive?

Oh, right: I'm a woman who was raised in a society that says there are very clear "right" and "wrong" ways to parent a child. And that those who choose to parent the "wrong" way are morally inferior, regardless of why they made that choice.

To the facilitator's credit, they responded to that mom with a gentle and nonjudgmental question: "Are you looking to change that?" To which the woman shook her head. The facilitator nodded, smiled, and moved on.

Seriously? They're not going to say something?

In hindsight, the black-and-white, vacuum-sealed nature of how proper infant care and safety advice is presented to pregnant women and new moms was undoubtedly one of the contributing factors to my intense anxiety.

Just like how "breast is best" for feeding, having a baby sleep alone in a crib may be the "best" option most of the time, but that advice doesn't account for what happens when a baby refuses to sleep independently in a crib.

Which is more dangerous: a new mom getting sleep stretches of at most 45 minutes at a time, or co-sleeping with the baby (using safe co-sleeping practices) and getting four hours at a time? I don't know—and that's my point.

Public health and medical professionals often present infant care and safety tips as if the answers about what's "best" are always straightforward. But the reality is that they're not, because context is everything. And context is constantly changing, even for the same family and the same baby.

For the record, I'm not recommending that people co-sleep with their baby. I'm merely suggesting that from a public health lens, there have been some unintended consequences of our hard-and-fast parenting "musts" in America: namely, deep and sometimes crippling anxiety among the rule-followers, as well as shame among those who choose a different path. Those very real consequences deserve some consideration.

Day after day, I slowly began buying into the group therapy model.

At the end of each week, we talked about our weekend plans. I remember one mom sharing her plans to meet up with friends.

We're allowed to do things like that?

At the time, I felt ashamed of what I was experiencing and thought I shouldn't be allowed to do "normal" things. My peers showed me that it was okay to continue on with life while battling mental illness.

Another mom talked about signing up for a running race for the fall. At first, I felt some excitement, because I used to run. But I hesitated, because it was only June, and up until that point I would've told you that I wasn't sure I would survive until the fall.

But I did it. I signed up. It was a quiet, personal, yet important act of faith that I would still be around in a few months.

I couldn't see it at the time, but that was where my recovery began. It began with each small act of bravery, each time that I carried on in spite of the deep fear and uncertainty I felt.

Early judgments aside, there was a strong sense of community among the women in that room, though we came from some very different backgrounds. We had a group text thread, and we sometimes continued conversations and jokes(!) that started in the therapy room. For example, a common concern among new moms—and not just those with severe mental health disorders—is whether or not a baby is pooping as often as they're "supposed" to be.

> **Hindsight note:** The range of normal when it comes to infant pooping schedules is actually shockingly wide.[17]

I found myself excitedly sharing news of my child's bowel movements with a group of strangers, some of whom I wouldn't have ever crossed paths with in the course of my everyday life.

Toward the end of my time in the program, I remember being counseled by one of the youngest mothers in the group that I would, eventually, be able to sit down with and truly enjoy a cup of coffee again. I'd previously shared that this was a feeling I feared was gone forever.

The act of lifting each other up in group therapy, and showering each other with the compassion and validation we had such a hard time offering ourselves, was a significant, and beautiful, part of the healing process.

I wish I could say that by the end of my four weeks in the program, I totally felt like "me" again, but that's not true. Truly feeling like "me" again took time and the utilization of many other supports, including (but not limited to) medication.

But the perinatal PHP reduced the severity of my symptoms and gave me a path forward. By the time I graduated, I was eating, I was sleeping, I had control over my bowels, and, perhaps most importantly, I knew that I wasn't alone.

This PHP was the lifeline that gave me the tools I needed for survival and helped me chart a path forward.

Zulresso (Brexanolone) Infusion

At my core, I'm a pretty happy person. I'm acutely aware of how good I have it in life, and I often mourn the passing of time. My biggest fear is death, because I love my life so much.

Although the perinatal PHP had gotten me through the worst of my experience, I knew deep down that something was still wrong. While I was no longer in acute agony (most of the time), I felt like I was now living in a meaningless, black-and-white world. That state of being was a far cry from normal for me, and that was painful and scary in itself. I could get out of bed, and I could even be convinced to do normal hobbies like baking or going for a bike ride with my husband, but it all felt flat.

Could this last forever? If it does, would I want to live like this forever?

While I wasn't in acute danger as I had been a few months prior, I was still struggling quite a bit, and I was willing to try every possible tool available to me to get "the real me" back.

So, a month or so later, I traveled out of state with my mom and Julian to receive an infusion treatment called Zulresso (generic name brexanolone). This was in 2023. At the time, Zulresso was the only medication specifically indicated and U.S. Food and Drug Administration (FDA)-approved for postpartum depression, and it had to be offered in an approved inpatient setting.[18] Unfortunately, it wasn't offered anywhere in my state.

This infusion treatment had come out in 2019, yet none of the providers I saw ever mentioned it. At my six-week postpartum visit with my primary OB, I told her I was looking into Zulresso and asked for her thoughts. She was vaguely supportive but admitted she didn't know much about it, and she advised that I should seek counsel from others before making a decision.

It was actually a Facebook group of about 500 moms who'd either received the infusion or were considering it that helped me learn about the treatment, the outcomes, and the process.

The scientific evidence was remarkable: studies had concluded that Zulresso infusion "provides prompt and effective resolution of depressive symptoms."[19] Considering that it often takes several months for the benefits of selective serotonin reuptake inhibitors (SSRIs), the most common pharmaceutical treatment for postpartum depression, to kick in, this statement is nothing short of amazing.

For a depressed new mother who's trying to care not only for herself but also for a vulnerable and highly impressionable infant each day, the value of "prompt" resolution of depressive symptoms cannot be overstated.

Having a master's degree in healthcare administration, a husband in medical school, and ample access to both healthcare and health insurance, yet learning about Zulresso—a highly effective, FDA-approved healthcare treatment for the *number one complication of childbirth*—through a Facebook group was a jarring experience. It took my trust in the U.S. healthcare system down several notches.

But because of that Facebook group, and because my insurance miraculously said that it would cover the treatment with no questions asked,[xiv] I took the leap and went for it. In that Facebook group, I saw stories that sounded like my own, but this time, they ended with miracle-like turnarounds rather than death and family heartbreak.

I wish I'd screenshotted some posts from that page, which no longer exists. It was a remarkable stockpile of awe-inducing personal stories of hope and recovery. It was also an amazing display of women from all walks of life stepping in to support other women, providing each other with hope and guidance to fill some of the gaps in our healthcare system.

I was excited to find this option, but I was also terrified of the glimmers of hope that it gave me.

How will it feel if I go all the way there, get this treatment, and still feel nothing? Will I still have the will to go on, or will the fear that I'll never feel like me again become too great?

For this reason, and because taking an eight-hour road trip with a twelve-week-old baby is a huge undertaking, we waffled at first.

---

xiv This is an enormous privilege that should not go unacknowledged; this is not the case for many women.

My husband, who was finishing up medical school, was skeptical. The medication came with a lot of warnings, including excessive sedation. And none of my doctors had known much about it, which, as an almost-physician himself, gave him pause.

But ultimately, in spite of our collective reservations, I decided that I wanted to give it a try. I wanted "my old brain" back, desperately.

———

Logistically, my experience of receiving the infusion was a great representation of the no-man's-land that exists between OB and psychiatric care.

Access to the Zulresso infusion, as evidenced by my need to travel out of state to receive it, was very limited. It feels important to reiterate the fact that several reports by this time had cited mental health conditions as the leading cause of maternal death, and that Zulresso was the only medication on the market specifically indicated for postpartum depression. But still, you could only receive this treatment in a finite number of locations.

One of the reasons for this was that it had to be given in an inpatient setting. This raised questions about many things, one of which was simply where to put the patient: psychiatry, OBGYN, or somewhere else? Most hospitals don't have perinatal psychiatric units. (More on that in Part 3.)

Due to visitor restrictions on psychiatric units, the out-of-state hospital I went to (thankfully) offered these infusions on an OBGYN unit.

For the three days I was in the hospital, it was abundantly clear that exceptions were being made for me to be on the unit receiving this care, and that the system was not designed for patients like me. I wasn't the typical OBGYN patient, and it showed.

Several times, nurses stopped by and asked if they could palpitate my uterus.

"Sure," I'd respond, "But I had my baby 12 weeks ago. I think my uterus is fine."

Another time, someone came in and congratulated me on my baby, then did a double take. "Wow, I've never seen such a big baby! C-section, I presume?" they said, thinking that I'd just birthed the three-month-old I was holding.

Yet another time, I had a young medical student (probably younger than me) try to counsel me about birth control options, with my mother sitting next to me.

"Thanks, but I've already had this exact conversation with my primary OB, six weeks ago. I'm good on that front."

Awkward and amusing experiences aside, this treatment, just like the perinatal PHP, was pivotal for me.

Going in, I'd prepared a long list of suggestions for myself about things to do or try if being confined to the bed inspired a bottomless panic attack again—a fear presumably rooted in my post-epidural childbirth experience. This list held things like:

- Call a friend
- Practice world geography on Sporcle
- Read a comedy book
- Join PSI support groups (I'd listed out several of their dates/times)
- And so on…

But to my astonishment, I was actually able to just relax in the bed, content to just exist or have a healthcare-related conversation with my aunt who visited me, since we both worked in healthcare administration.

Sleep came and went fairly easily to me (!!!), even if I was awoken in the night. On day two, I pulled out my computer and began chipping away at the script for the wedding I'd been asked to officiate later that summer, which until that moment I hadn't been sure I was going to be able to do.

And by the end of the two-and-a-half-day infusion, I was laughing—really, genuinely, laughing—at comedy specials on Netflix with my mom, which was something I hadn't been able to do since before Julian was born.

I was also initiating wholesome conversations like, "I wonder what kind of routines I could implement with Julian to give him the best chance of avoiding anxiety and depression when he's older. Maybe we should add talking about something we're grateful for to his bedtime routine so it becomes a habit," and I'd made a mental note to do more research on that topic later.[xv]

A few weeks after my infusion, I was back at work, and a few weeks after that, I flew down to Colorado (Julian in tow!) to officiate that wedding. A few months later, I took the plunge and started coaching gymnastics, my first love, part-time: something I'd been itching to do since the sport imploded in 2016[xvi] and revealed a desperate need for coaches who genuinely care about the health and well-being of children.

The "real" me was back, and arguably better than before, despite carrying some serious emotional battle wounds.

---

xv   Remember, my child was all of 12 weeks old at the time. Daily gratitude rituals weren't what he needed for his mental health; he mostly just needed *me* to have strong mental health.

xvi   If this doesn't mean anything to you, Google "Larry Nassar."

To be clear, I was (and still am) on medication and in regular therapy. However, at this point in my journey, mental health recovery became just one piece of my life, not the defining feature of it.

At some point, as I began reflecting on my journey, my ever-the-businessman dad heard me talking about how grateful I was for the perinatal PHP. He asked me, "I thought you said it was the infusion that made you feel better. Which was it, the hospital program or the infusion?"

I love my family dearly, but let's just say mental health isn't our strongest subject. In our family, positivity is expected, sadness is to be avoided, and anger and frustration are regarded as character flaws. Low motivation is evidence of laziness: one of the worst characteristics of all and worthy of contempt.

To him, I'd clearly been ill, and somebody had "fixed" me. Who did it; who got the credit? Which "product" worked?

So, I want to be clear: there's no "or" in this situation, and nobody "fixed" me, because I was never broken. My illness was the result of a perfect storm: the abrupt drop in hormones from childbirth, learned fear and rejection of negative emotions, deeply etched perfectionism, internalized messages from living in a society that expects the world of yet offers little to mothers, and perhaps some personal brain chemistry issues, among other factors.

Mental health disorders aren't (typically) like a broken arm in need of surgery; they're more like diabetes or other chronic conditions that are multifactorial in both their causes and their treatments. I healed so quickly and so completely because in the end, I was able to access so many different, and complementary, resources.

So, I'm unbelievably grateful that I was able to access both the perinatal PHP *and* the Zulresso infusion. Both of those resources played an important—and distinct—role in my recovery, as did significant levels of family support, a kind and generous peer support mentor, free online support groups through PSI, and tried-and-true good nutrition, exercise, and sleep.

All that said, the perinatal PHP was undoubtedly the single most critical part of my recovery. It was the source of my insight into my condition, and it quickly became my medical "home" for all things related to my reproductive mental health. It connected me with a handful of other women who became lifelines well past discharge. Without having a qualified team who could help me navigate my symptoms, my perceptions of myself, and my treatment plans, I wouldn't be where I am today.

In a surge of gratitude one evening, about a year and half after my story unfolded, I sat down and wrote a letter of support for the Other Local Health System PHP, in case something like that could be useful to them. I knew enough about healthcare funding to know that programs like this are often supported by philanthropy, and that philanthropy is largely driven by storytelling.

The last line in that letter was: "I wish every new mom suffering from postpartum depression or anxiety had access to a program like [perinatal PHP] to help them navigate the darkness and uncertainty."

And then it hit me.

What if I could use my story to help make that a reality?

And so it began: my relentless quest for change.

PART 2

Advocating From Within

Before We Begin...

What I really wanted to do with this section was include full, unedited emails between me and the leaders of Large Nonprofit Health System. And if not full, then paraphrased. I wanted to show you, rather than tell you, *exactly* how hard I fought for simple changes to be made for moms and babies, to leave no room for assumptions regarding what was, or wasn't, said.

But I'm not going to.

Partly because the more time goes on, and the more I learn about the state of women's healthcare in the U.S., the less all of the specific conversations matter to me.

But mostly, it's because I've been advised to tread ~extraordinarily~ carefully, since I'm critiquing a powerful organization within a powerful industry. So, instead, I'm recalling my experiences from memory and sharing recollections of only the most impactful conversations that I had.

Before we begin, therefore, I have a request. If at any point you find yourself thinking, "Huh—she must not have been clear or direct enough," or perhaps, "Hmm—she must not have been kind or respectful enough," just make a mental note of it, and maybe start a tally.

I ask this because along my journey, I've conveyed my profound disappointment in Large Nonprofit Health System leaders to many people in my personal and professional circles. Several, from my father to seasoned healthcare industry veterans, have responded something along those lines.

I can only assume that this is because the concept of good people in positions of power looking the other way and/or choosing to do nothing when presented with concrete information about how to save the lives of new moms seemed too absurd for them to comprehend, too.

It's far easier (again, presumably) to assume that I—a young woman—failed to do things The Right Way.

"Too docile, maybe? Too direct, perhaps? Maybe she didn't cite her sources. Or she didn't convey, "I'm a team player" well enough? Nobody likes a hostile young person."

I invite you to notice if, and when, you make these assumptions, and to try to give me the benefit of the doubt. I was ready to include more detailed information here, because I'm confident in how I went about things. But at the same time, I put a high priority on protecting my peace, and I've learned not to assume *anything* about what people in positions of power will or will not do to protect themselves.

Chip on my shoulder aside, make no mistake: **what happened to me at Large Nonprofit Health System could have happened to me at any health system across the United States**. Don't assume that your local health system would never respond the way that Large Nonprofit Health System leaders responded to me. If that were true, we probably wouldn't be in the position we are today, where maternal mental health disorders are the leading cause of maternal mortality, and high-quality, specialized care is nearly impossible to access.

Disclaimer: All names and personal identifiers have been changed, and the interactions I discuss in this section are reflections of the personal experiences I had trying to advocate for improvements. Conversations are reconstructed the way I remember them, to the best of my memory.

CHAPTER 6

Before the Fight

Who Am I?

At the risk of sounding like an insufferably arrogant young woman, I'd like to back up and give you some context about what my professional role was at the time of this experience, and why I was so naively confident that speaking up would lead to positive, meaningful change.

After a couple of years as a healthcare consultant after college, I went back to graduate school and earned my Master's of Healthcare Administration (MHA) from a well-established, highly ranked MHA program.

Throughout the program, we had guest lectures by practicing healthcare executives from all over the country, all imparting the same general message to me and my classmates: "Our healthcare system needs you. Go out and change the world. Take risks. Healthcare is in good hands because of ambitious and mission-driven young people like you."

I, like many of my classmates, took this guidance to heart and, with each and every assignment, tried to put it into practice.

By the end of my graduate program, I'd racked up a handful of accolades that reflected my ability to take in information, process it, and make thoughtful recommendations about how to address a given problem.

I won a national essay contest by writing about the promise of Hospital at Home programs, which shortly afterward saw an explosion of popularity. The explosion in popularity was not by any stretch of the imagination the result of my essay, though it *was* an indication that I did indeed have a clue what I was talking about when arguing that such programs were a valid solution to a pressing healthcare crisis.

I won multiple case competitions, one of which involved flying to another state with a few of my classmates to deliver a 15-minute presentation to executives of a Fortune 5 company. Another involved making sense of a massive, public, raw healthcare data file and producing a presentation with meaningful insights in just one weekend.

I won a prestigious health policy scholarship, which in non-COVID times would have included an all-expenses-paid trip to D.C. to meet with policymakers.

After graduation, I joined Large Nonprofit Health System. It was a health system that seemed highly regarded among alumni and that, on paper, was aligned with everything I stood for in healthcare: improving quality, improving patient and provider experience, and decreasing costs (aka the Quadruple Aim).[20]

I was an administrative fellow, which meant I reported directly to senior leaders, worked on a wide range of projects, and had a lot of face time with those in the C-suite. Through this position, I had the privilege of working with and getting to know several senior leaders at Large Nonprofit Health System, many of whom I deeply respected and admired.

By all accounts, I did well during my fellowship. I was routinely praised for my reliability, my collaboration skills, my critical thinking, and my integrity.

On top of all this, I'd developed what I thought were strong personal relationships with several of the senior leaders at Large Nonprofit Health System. One of them generously offered me an entire car-load of hand-me-downs for my son when I was pregnant, which I very gratefully accepted.

All this is to say that, after everything I went through in my tumultuous postpartum period, I was sure, *absolutely sure*, that the people I'd worked with—the people at or near the head of Large Nonprofit Health System—would be furious *with* me about what had happened during my postpartum period and ready to rectify the gaps in care that I'd experienced. Not simply to right a past wrong, but to save the next woman from going through some of the avoidable pain and suffering that I did.

In retrospect, I was astonishingly naive.

Sometimes, I look back at that sweet, younger version of myself and feel embarrassed, given how things played out in the end.

*How silly must I have looked, sharing vulnerable details
of my life and expecting them to take action as a result?
Did they roll their eyes after each email or meeting?*

But on the bright side, my naivety meant that I went into my advocacy efforts at Large Nonprofit Health System with the purest of intentions. After all, I really thought we were on the same team.

It took me about a year and a half to realize that maybe, in fact, we weren't.

The names and genders of everyone involved have been changed to protect their privacy, and some individuals are simply referred to as Leaders A–D. I've also omitted specific titles and departments, though I hope you'll trust me when I say I raised these issues with the people in leadership positions whom I believed were most likely to be able to enact change.

You'll also see time stamps; these are anchored on the day I first shared my personal experience and concerns with a senior leader at Large Nonprofit Health System, which I refer to as "Day 0." Time stamps are approximate.

Returning to Work

Following my maternity leave, my plan had been to transition to a new team within Large Nonprofit Health System, as is common at the end of an administrative fellowship.

I was excited about my new role; it was truly my dream job, at least for that stage of my career and my life. My new role was on a small team, doing the exact kind of work I love to do, and with the kind of flexibility that might actually allow me to keep my head above water with a one-year-old and a husband working long hours in residency (if such a thing is possible). And it paid well enough to help us comfortably afford childcare, which, as any new parent in the U.S. knows, is not a given. It was a win on all fronts.

But in the thick of my postpartum struggle, I started to doubt whether starting this new job as planned was going to be feasible after all.

I can barely handle the stress of simply existing as a new mom. How can I possibly add work on top of that? Besides, something happened to my brain. It isn't the same as it used to be. Am I even capable of this work anymore? What if I do a terrible job and get fired?

I reached out immediately to some of the leaders in my network, including my new boss. I felt awful about letting anyone down,[xvii] because a lot of people had advocated for me and advised me along my post-fellowship job search and transition process.

When I spoke with my soon-to-be boss Deb, they were kind, generous, and compassionate. They stressed that we could change my start date, change my work schedule, and in general do *whatever I needed* to navigate the transition back. It was the dream response, and I was—and forever will be—so grateful.

All of this validated my gut instinct that yes, of course I wanted to go back to work, and no, I didn't hold Large Nonprofit Health System or any of its leaders personally responsible for the many process failures that had so recently led me down a path to suicidal ideation, inpatient hospitalization, and a world of hurt.

These are really good people. They must just have no idea how many gaps there are in the system for new moms. Just imagine what we can do and how much we can change once I share my experience with them and offer to help!

Largely due to the miracle of Zulresso, I started my new role nearly on time as planned, though I took my boss up on their offer of having me start part-time.

An Awkward Encounter (The First of Many)

One of those first few days in the office, one of my new co-workers said, "Wow! You look great! I can hardly tell you had a baby a few months ago."

---

xvii Sensing a pattern here, anyone?

It caught me off guard, and I didn't know what to say.

Unfortunately, I went with something along the lines of, "Thanks—I had really bad anxiety and depression. I couldn't really eat for most of that time."

Tremendous awkwardness ensued. I still cringe thinking about it.

It wasn't my intention to make her feel bad. I was just one of those new moms navigating the often-awkward transition back to work and "the real world" after spending several months under a rock while home with a baby. And add to my journey an immense amount of trauma, which rendered almost all "Welcome back!" and "Congratulations!" platitudes a little bit painful and confusing to respond to, even if they were offered with good intentions.

CHAPTER 7

Day 0

The Conversations Begin

A few months into my new role, I worked up the courage to reach out to Leader A, a high-ranking leader whom I knew quite well from my time as an administrative fellow. I asked if they'd be willing to connect virtually, which they happily agreed to.

Great! This is a good sign.

In that short meeting, I shared with them a brief summary of what had happened, how I ultimately climbed out of the deep, dark hole I'd been in, and a few of the areas I thought we could improve as a care system.

Though the conversation went okay, I sensed right away that Leader A was more interested in offering sympathy for a difficult experience and less interested in hearing my thoughts on ways we could improve. To be on the safe side, and to drive home some tangible next steps, I sent them a follow-up message that both expressed gratitude for the conversation and reiterated some key points.

One of those key points was around our postpartum depression screening process. As you may recall from Part 1, my experience of being screened for postpartum depression actually *escalated* my symptoms, because it didn't lead me to the help I needed in a timely manner. Instead, my disclosure of thoughts of suicide resulted in an offer of a one-hour virtual therapy appointment in one week's time: something I thought reflected a complete misunderstanding of what was happening.

I stressed in my early conversations with Leader A that we should review the screening process to ensure that any and all providers who conducted postpartum depression screenings were equipped to respond appropriately if and when they identified a woman in crisis.

Instead of agreeing that ensuring timely and adequate response was of the utmost importance, they noted that this "issue" was already on their radar, and already taken care of.

I was told that we now followed up on all positive screens, because someone else had already spoken up about the fact that for some amount of time, we *were not always following up on positive screens.*

This revealed something deeply alarming about the state of our standard processes.

My point about the depression screenings had been that the follow-up to my positive screen was woefully inadequate, thus making me feel much worse and more hopeless than I had been going into the appointment. Emphasis on the quality and content of the follow-up… assuming the *existence* of the follow-up itself was a given.

*You used to just… **not respond** to "positive screens"? Holy shit; that's even worse.*

Leader A's response revealed to me that, until recently, it had been commonplace for women to fill out a postpartum depression screening, disclose thoughts of self-harm or suicide, and then not receive *any* kind of follow-up.

Can you imagine how devastating that must have been for those moms, who bravely answered that screening form honestly, presumably thinking it would lead to help of some kind—only to be left hanging, without even a courtesy phone call?

Yikes.

Yikes yikes yikes.

Always Lead With Positivity

I am solutions-oriented, arguably to a fault.

Growing up under the influence of a successful, conservative, white male businessman father and a white, no-nonsense tiger mom, I've always implicitly understood that the best (and only?) way for me to initiate change—in anything—is to somehow be clear, direct, and well-researched while simultaneously being *exceedingly* gracious and agreeable. I knew that those who come off as "too angry" are dismissed by people in positions of power almost immediately.

So, I did my best with this implicit assignment, while at the same time reeling about the rapidly growing hill I had to climb ahead of me.

I respectfully acknowledged the "progress" that Leader A had shared with me, but I reiterated my feedback that *how* we responded in those moments of crisis mattered quite a bit.

In these early conversations, I also acknowledged (and cited) that mental health conditions are now the most common cause of pregnancy-related death in the U.S., and that my own experience had helped me see why that might be the case. I shared specific, free resources that our providers could leverage as needed, and I consistently volunteered to be of help on that topic in any way, at any time, for the sake of future moms.

And I *always* tried to conclude on a note of positivity, typically emphasizing the "significant opportunity ahead" rather than what we had maybe been doing poorly in the past.

CHAPTER 8

Day 15

A Significant Advancement in the Field

A couple of weeks after those initial conversations, there was a significant milestone in postpartum depression treatment. The company that made Zulresso had launched a new drug called Zurzuvae (generic name zuranolone), which was similar to Zulresso but an oral formulation. This meant it would be far more accessible than its predecessor, which required inpatient hospitalization.[21]

I used this occasion as an excuse to circle back with Leader A on the topic of maternal mental health, as our exchanges had seemed to fizzle out.

I reached out with (genuine!) excitement, letting them know about this important new development and where to find more information about it if needed.

Given that a few weeks had passed without any further discussion or action on a subject that I knew to be quite literally life-or-death for some number of moms, I'd started to suspect that maybe Leader A hadn't fully grasped the gravity of what I'd been sharing.

So, I shared a short CBS clip[22] that had just aired regarding the new treatment. In the segment, Joy Burkhard,

CEO and Founder of the Policy Center for Maternal Mental Health, talked with a reporter about the accountability gap in U.S. healthcare that allows women to slip through the cracks when neither OB/midwife, primary care, or psychiatry really wants to take "ownership" of a postpartum mother with mental health concerns. I'd experienced that kind of disheartening provider ping-pong game personally, so it was one of the key issues I wanted to bring to Leader A's attention.

Leader A thanked me for sharing the information, and quickly assured me that they felt we were well positioned to ensure that women *didn't* fall through the cracks.

Sure… but we're not executing on that potential, obviously.

This conversation is even more painful in hindsight, because just a few months later, we did in fact lose another mom to "the cracks." (More on that later.)

CHAPTER 9

Day 35

Thanks, But No Thanks

A few weeks later, I had the chance to talk with a couple more leaders about both my experience and the FDA approval of Zurzuvae. They were kind, but nothing of substance (to my knowledge) came from the interaction.

Each person I met offered sympathy for the experience I'd endured and assured me that such a thing would never happen again, for fill-in-the-blank highly specific reason. Collectively, from my perspective, these well-meaning leaders were gaslighting me (and perhaps themselves) into thinking that the epic problem I *thought* existed was actually a simple one that had, in fact, been rectified already.

Shortly afterward, I had one last conversation with Leader A. It was a conversation that, in my opinion, quietly solidified that I was not to be part of the ongoing improvement team on this topic (if one existed).

Leader A reached out, unprompted, and thanked me again for sharing my feedback with the team. But, instead of thoughtful dialogue that continued an important conversation, it felt vaguely like a form rejection email you might get after a job interview: polite, but firmly saying, "Thanks, but no thanks."

I was crushed.

I had worked with this particular leader up until the day I went on maternity leave.

To me, their final message to me came across as: "I have taken the obligatory amount of time to humor you, and now this conversation is over."

It also framed all of my comments and insights as simply patient feedback rather than the insights of a qualified health-care leader with lived experience, which is what I believed I was really offering.

Hitting My Limit

This last conversation brought my internal advocacy efforts to a grinding halt, temporarily.

Here I was, sharing highly vulnerable yet critically important and time-sensitive feedback with someone I believed had the power to actually do something about it. But they were gently, yet firmly, closing our line of communication on the subject.

To say I was disappointed would be an understatement. I also felt betrayed, frustrated, angry, and deeply worried about the implications of this outcome. I felt levels of fear, grief, and insecurity that I hadn't felt since the depth of my illness: feelings that I still wasn't comfortable sitting with.

Fortunately, by this point, I'd developed more self-awareness about the state of my mental health. A quick self-assessment of my emotional state showed me that while I was ready to share what had happened to me, I didn't yet feel ready to hold the weight of indifference.[xviii]

[xviii] Though fortunately, that strength would later come, as I've now learned that holding the weight of indifference is an inextricable aspect of being an advocate for anything important.

I knew that I wanted to speak up for the women behind me and to change the system that had failed me and others so badly. But I also knew that, above all, I needed to care for myself, if for no other reason than because I also now understood that would be best for my baby.

So, after that conversation, I took an intentional pause on advocating for maternal mental health improvements within Large Nonprofit Health System.

After wiping my tears and collecting myself, I sent a brief response, making sure to express my gratitude once more and end on a note of continued optimism, even though I no longer felt that way inside.

Throughout the entire "phase 1" of my advocacy process, I felt that I was never viewed as a colleague with valuable experience that should inform continued improvement efforts; rather, I was treated strictly as a patient sharing a run-of-the-mill patient complaint.

And clearly, once again, from my perspective, there seemed to be a process for handling such things: hear them out, assure them that you're already on top of it, and escort them out the door.

CHAPTER 10

Day 150

Celebrating Maternal Mental Health Awareness Month

As Julian's first birthday approached, I realized that I was ready to start sharing my story more publicly, even if I wasn't ready to resume any more conversations about it within Large Nonprofit Health System. Despite the frustrating experience with advocacy, I was really enjoying my new role on Deb's team. I was allowing myself some time to breathe and just focus on continuing to build my reputation as a hard-working, insightful, competent emerging leader.

I first shared my story on social media in honor of Maternal Mental Health Month. This gave me a surge of confidence, because it was met with many kind responses and validation from my personal and professional networks alike.

Using some of this confidence, I made the decision to share some timely maternal health information with some of the leaders I'd spoken with a few months prior. Our state health department had recently sent out information about the national Centers for Disease Control and Prevention (CDC) "Hear Her" campaign,[23] which included free educational materials that could be used by healthcare organizations like ours.

I figured that the leaders probably (hopefully?) knew of this campaign already, given its direct relevance to their work, but I decided to err on the side of caution in case they didn't.

The responses I received were kind, but they gave me the impression that the leaders were not already familiar with this campaign and these resources provided by our state health department. This was slightly unsettling, given that Large Nonprofit Health System was one of the major providers of prenatal and delivery care in our large metro area.

Not a huge deal, just another minor disappointment to add to my ever-growing pile.

I'm not sure whether or not this information *actually* got shared with any of Large Nonprofit Health System's patients or providers, but if it did, I certainly never heard about it.

After that brief intermission, I returned to my hidey-hole, and I stayed there awhile.

CHAPTER 11

Day 350+

A Chance Encounter

Roughly six months later, I went to a healthcare networking event. One of the panelists at the event was the CEO of Other Local Health System: the health system that runs the perinatal PHP that I credit with saving my life.

After the event, I waited in a long line to introduce myself to the CEO. I wanted to personally thank them for supporting a program that I knew from my professional expertise was probably not profitable or straightforward to sustain.

It was worth the wait: they were kind, compassionate, and refreshingly transparent. They hugged me, thanked me for sharing, and validated that maternal mental health is an overlooked and under-resourced issue. They confirmed that supporting the perinatal PHP was difficult and let me in on a fact that shook me to my core: that they struggled with utilization of the program.

Let's pause there for a moment.

DEMAND

Somewhere between 50,000 and 100,000 babies are born each year in the state in which I live (I'm keeping this intentionally broad, because this is simply an order of magnitude demonstration).

Roughly 20% of the women who give birth to those babies likely suffer from a perinatal mental health disorder, of which I will (very) conservatively estimate that 10% are severe enough to warrant intensive treatment.

Using some basic arithmetic:

75,000 births per year (midpoint of the range stated above) × 20% prevalence × 10% severe = ~**1,500 women/year in need of intensive care**

There are only eight seats (aka "beds") in the perinatal PHP program, and most of the women I encountered attended for four weeks.

CAPACITY

8 beds × 4 days/week × 52 weeks/year = 1,664 "bed-days" per year

Most women attending for four weeks means that most women use 16 bed-days.

1,664 bed-days available / 16 bed-days needed per patient = **maximum capacity of 104 women/year**

SO WHAT?

My point here is that if Other Local Health System was struggling to fill their perinatal PHP—the only one in the entire state—it wasn't due to lack of need. It was due to lack of awareness, lack of appropriate referrals, and/or lack of ability to access this kind of care.

I couldn't believe what I was hearing.

By this point, it had been nearly a year since I'd pleaded directly with those near the top of Large Nonprofit Health System to educate our relevant providers about the existence of the nearby perinatal PHP, build some sort of direct referral pathway to that program for women with severe symptoms, or *at the very least* reference that program on our website. Yet none of that had happened, and here I was, hearing that the life-saving, resource-intensive program was struggling with utilization.

I was sad on behalf of all the mothers in the preceding year who should have been directed to the perinatal PHP, which was an incredible resource available in only a handful of cities across the country. Given the well-established statistics about the prevalence of perinatal mental health disorders, I knew this meant that many women who could have been better served by the perinatal PHP had been white-knuckling it at home or in an inpatient psychiatric unit without their child.

But on an even deeper level, I was terrified about the implications of that statement in a tenuous financial environment in healthcare.

What will happen if there are substantial budget cuts in the future? Could someone (say, a young male consultant, perhaps?) look at the utilization of the program, conclude that there's insufficient demand and that the benefits of the program don't justify the cost, and close it?

That thought terrified me, and it spurred me right back into action.

Bringing It Back to Large Nonprofit Health System

The next week, I asked Deb if they would be okay with me spending some time working on an overview of maternal mental healthcare. I proposed putting together a summary of the gaps in our system as well as gaps in the local market that I knew about based on my own experience and my subsequent research.

Without much, if any, hesitation, they agreed. I proceeded to spend a few days putting together a slide deck that neatly summarized what I'd experienced, what I'd learned, and what I thought we ought to be doing in light of all of that.

This deck reiterated some of what I'd discussed with Leader A and other leaders a year prior, but it was now more cleanly packaged and presented, and it included receipts: screenshots from my medical records that verified that I was not, unfortunately, exaggerating in my recollection of what had transpired.

When I was ready to share that slide deck, and with a thumbs-up from Deb, I sent a meeting invitation and a corresponding email to Deb, Leader A, and Leader B (another high-ranking, relevant leader). I gave them a heads-up that the last few slides contained personal details about my experience and clarified that I'd redacted all provider names, because my goal was to highlight systemic issues, not to critique any individual providers.

This is true, was true, and will always be true.

Yet Another Disappointing Conversation

Around the same time that I sent my presentation to this small group of leaders, I sent an update to the few others to whom I'd spoken the first time around. Of course, my update included gratitude, and it also emphasized my desire to listen and learn about any changes that I should be aware of since our last conversation.

Shortly thereafter, I found myself in another meeting in which—as I should have come to expect—we spent most of the time with someone explaining to me how and why what I *thought* was still a problem was, in fact, no longer a significant problem.

During our conversation, this person repeatedly referred to the PHP I'd attended as an intensive outpatient program (IOP), which, as I'll discuss more in Chapter 22, is a similar but meaningfully different level of care.

At one point, I asked their opinion about whether a specialized inpatient unit for perinatal women was necessary or should be an advocacy priority, or whether they thought that *with proper utilization and perhaps growth of new and existing outpatient programs*, we could avoid the need for a perinatal inpatient unit altogether.

Their response? No, they didn't think a specialized inpatient unit in our state was necessary, because "women that severe" could simply be admitted to a general adult inpatient unit.

That was it: no questions for me, and no evident curiosity about my opinion on that statement as someone who'd openly been one of "those severe cases" sent to a general inpatient unit in the recent past. Just a quick dismissal of the concept that we could or should concern ourselves with how we're caring for the sickest new mothers and their families and whether we could do any better. (More on this in Chapter 22.)

The incomplete grasp of treatment levels for maternal mental health and the lack of humility demonstrated by this individual's responses were profound. And this wasn't just anybody at Large Nonprofit Health System; this was one of the relevant clinical leaders.

Yikes. On a macro level, I think I might know more about this topic than they do. This is not a good sign.

Momentum Waxes...

A few days later, I received a surprisingly encouraging response from Leader A regarding the email, calendar invite, and presentation I'd shared with them, Leader B, and Deb.

Great! Maybe we're on the same page now. Maybe my timing was just bad, but now the timing is better and they're ready to partner with me on this.

Feeling emboldened by Leader A's response, I reached out to Leader C, another high-ranking leader in our organization and someone with whom I was fortunate enough to have a pre-existing relationship through prior project work. I admired their accessible, down-to-earth leadership style and their (seemingly) genuine commitment to the well-being of both our patients and our care teams, and I figured they'd be interested in this conversation. I wanted to loop them into these conversations, because I was hopeful they might be willing to champion improvement efforts and prioritization of the issue.

The next day, I received a very kind and enthusiastic response, which was precisely what I'd come to expect from Leader C.

I shared the materials I'd already shared with my boss, Leader A, and Leader B.

Then, as tends to be the case in corporate America in mid to late December, progress took a hiatus until the new year.

...And Momentum Wanes

Reschedule #1 of my meeting with Deb, Leader A, and Leader B. No notes provided, just an updated calendar request.

*No problem. I should have known better than to sched-
ule a meeting in late December when nobody cares about
anything they're not legally required to immediately care
about. My bad.*

Reschedule #2.

I was disappointed, but I understood that things come up
and that priorities are constantly shifting. So, I responded with
a message saying I would be happy to meet in a few weeks.

Putting an Innovation Lesson Into Practice

Around the same time that all of this was happening, I received an invitation to share my personal story at a large maternal mental health conference in D.C. hosted by the Policy
Center for Maternal Mental Health. While the prospect was
daunting, I knew that by sharing my story, I could help other
moms, so I eagerly said yes.

About three months prior, I'd attended a mandatory meeting at Large Nonprofit Health System centered around the
topic of innovation. It was fantastic.

One of the tools we learned about was starting any new
project by writing a fictional future press release. "Write from
a future perspective," the facilitator suggested. "Write about
what you hope to be true by the time you're done. Then work
backward to figure out how to get there."

That meeting resonated with me on many levels, because
I'm passionate about the need for innovation in healthcare and
interested in learning how to foster innovative thinking both
in myself and in others.

As I was writing the draft of my speech for the upcoming conference, I had an epiphany: "I should conclude this draft with *what I hope to be true by the time I give the talk.* I will share not just my patient story but also what Large Nonprofit Health System did in response to my story: what actions *we* took that other health systems can learn from."

So, that's precisely what I did. I dreamed up my ideal conclusion to share with the conference audience, one that would demonstrate what it looks like for a large health system to take meaningful steps forward in light of the information at hand. The end of my first draft read as follows:

> "The Policy Center for Maternal Mental Health has a survey of best practices that both hospitals and insurers can take to evaluate how well their systems are set up to support the mental health of new moms and what actions they should take to improve.
>
> The organization that I work for, Large Nonprofit Health System, has committed to using this survey as a starting point for addressing gaps in our health system, and we have already begun making changes. My ask today is for other organizations to do the same."

I was fully prepared to go to this conference and hype up Large Nonprofit Health System as a leader in this space, not just in maternal mental health but in the act of seeing, appreciating, and acting on difficult patient safety feedback.

Now, all I had to do was work backward and make those statements a reality.

CHAPTER 12

Days 410+

The Conversation I'd Been Dreaming Of...

My conversation with Leader C occurred around Day 410, and it was nothing short of amazing.

I accidentally caught them off guard with a deeply raw and provocative essay about my experience, which they read in real time, because they hadn't seen it come through their inbox the day prior.

My essay began with a hypothetical: one where I hadn't survived my mental health crisis.

It went on to offer a description (through rose-colored glasses) of what might have happened as a result, knowing that tragedy often spurs people—at least temporarily—into action. It concluded by challenging our leaders to act with as much urgency as they might have if I'd died: to not be complacent simply because I'd happened to survive.

I had the privilege of watching their real-time processing and reactions to what I was sharing, which was *everything I'd hoped and expected it might be.*

I'm paraphrasing, but our conversation, as I recall it, went something like this:

Leader C: "Wow. Thank you so much for bringing this to me."

Me: "Thank *you* so much for your willingness to hear my story and talk with me about this. I wasn't sure if it was appropriate to reach out to you directly, but I've always admired your leadership and found you approachable."

Leader C: "Please don't worry about bringing something like this directly to me—I *need* to know things like this."

I told them about how, when I'd been in group therapy, I'd felt responsible for the healthcare process failures experienced by the women around me. I was all of 27 at the time—hardly responsible for anything yet, professionally speaking—but I had an MHA and was proud of my profession. So, sitting in a room full of women who'd experienced many of the same process gaps that I had filled me with shame.

"It's funny that you used that phrase, 'I felt so responsible.' Because that's how I felt when I read your essay," Leader C said to me. "How can we make this better? How can I be most helpful?"

I responded something to this effect: "The most helpful thing you could do for me would be to reiterate to others in leadership that this is an opportunity for quality improvement. I'm worried that others do not or will not want me to speak about this so openly, but if you see this as a clear opportunity for improvement the way I do and would be willing to vouch for that, I'd really appreciate it."

"Of course," they said. "And absolutely continue to tell your story. It's important."

They continued, without any prompting whatsoever, along the lines of the following:

"You have always stood out among young leaders in our organization. I hope you make your career here with us. Not just your current role, but future roles too. We need people like you."

I left their office on cloud nine.

Yes! I knew it! They're a great leader, and they see the improvement and industry leadership opportunity here that I see. And they have the clout to get it prioritized. It's going to happen.

I sent several messages to people in my inner circle saying things like, "Just met with Leader C. It went AMAZING!!!!!"

... Followed by Deafening Silence

Like always, I sent a thoughtful follow-up email a day or two after the meeting.

I never got a response.

Given how unequivocally positive our one-on-one conversation had seemed, this surprised me.

My frustration was mounting, along with my concern about whether or not I was being taken seriously. Over the weekend, I got a response from a popular healthcare blog that I'd reached out to about publishing the same essay I'd just shown Leader C. They said they would be happy to publish it.

I was thrilled but conflicted. I still hadn't heard anything back from Leader C. They'd encouraged me to tell my story and hadn't expressed any concerns with the essay when they read it, but still, I knew it might ruffle feathers, and the last thing I wanted was to blindside them. I considered them my ally, so I wanted to make sure they really supported me going public with that essay.

I reached out, and they offered to talk to me for a few minutes by phone.

On the phone, they seemed distant. Maybe they were just distracted by other priorities, or maybe they were now intentionally pulling back a little bit.

I let them know that I'd found an outlet that was interested in publishing the essay we'd discussed the week before, and that I was planning to move forward.

"Like I said before, I never want to get in the way of you telling your story," they said.

I hung up the phone, and I gave the blog a thumbs-up.

***

Reschedule #3 for the meeting with Leader A, Leader B, and Deb. No explanation.

***

Reschedule #4. No explanation.

The Essay Goes Public

Over 400 days from when I'd first raised my concerns about the gaps in our care process for new moms, and nearly two weeks after I'd had previewed this same essay with Leader C, my first public blog post about my experience with postpartum anxiety and depression was published.

It included all of the ways in which my health system had failed to intervene, and all of the things I wished they'd done in response. It even acknowledged that the lack of urgency around the issue was an ongoing trauma of its own.

They will reach out. They will read it and say something like, "Oh my goodness, I didn't realize it was SO bad. I'm sorry we didn't take you seriously sooner. That was a mistake. Let's fix this."

I shared the post on LinkedIn and my personal social media, and, similar to when I'd posted in honor of Maternal Mental Health Month, I got an immediate flood of support, validation, and gratitude from people in my personal and professional networks.

An acquaintance from college who was now a practicing physician said, "Thank you for sharing your story. I just wanted to reach out and say that as someone who cares for pregnant and postpartum patients every day, your words really impacted me, and your story will absolutely inform how I approach my patients for the rest of my career."

But from the leaders within my own organization, at whom this essay was directed, I heard nothing. Enough people at my organization interacted with the post that I knew *with certainty* that it had crossed my leaders' radars.

But I received no calls, no emails, no instant messages, no comments.

Nothing.

After sharing such a vulnerable post with the world—one that I'd so diligently previewed with one of our highest leaders, who'd given me their verbal support—the silence was more than disappointing. It was humiliating.

Was I just imagining that they ever cared about me or that they ever believed in my leadership potential?

By this point, it had been over two weeks since my meeting with Leader C, the one where I walked out beaming, sure that I'd found just the right ally: someone with integrity, an eye for quality improvement opportunities, and the clout to move things along.

Not only had they not followed up in any way or responded to my email, but they also hadn't acknowledged that the gut-punching essay I'd previewed with them had now been swirling on the internet for days.

And with that, the hope that I'd been holding for so long— that *somehow, in some way* I'd be able to get Large Nonprofit Health System to act—began to fade.

CHAPTER 13

Day 435

Where Is the Urgency?

One week later.

Still, nobody had reached out to me (good or bad) about the blog post. After being rescheduled several times over six weeks, my short meeting with Deb, Leader A, and Leader B was just a few days away.

But given the abrupt silence, the constant rescheduling, and the short duration of time we had on the calendar, I knew things weren't looking good. Their silence in the preceding weeks had already told me which direction this was heading, and it was not a promising one.

I was sitting at my desk, and I suddenly felt the need to pull out a notebook and write. This is what came out:

Urgency (Or Lack Thereof)

It almost killed me then.
It's killing others now.
I've presented you with solutions.

Specific.

Reasonable.
Actionable.

And you've presented me with silence.

Silence that tells me everything I need to know about the value you place on the life of a woman.

A woman like me.
A woman like you.
A woman like her.

A Last-Ditch Effort

With the writing on the wall that Large Nonprofit Health System was choosing silence over action, I decided to throw a Hail Mary.

One of the only people at the top of the organization whom I'd not yet spoken with about this topic was another high-ranking leader, Leader D.

Once again, this was someone I had a strong relationship with already. Leader D was a role model to me and an advocate of mine. I'd waited a long time to loop them into this conversation out of respect for their position and a desire to avoid abusing my relationship with someone who held such significant influence.

Again, I wish I could share the email verbatim, because I still stand behind it today.

But legally, I can't.

So, I'll just leave it at this: the email I sent to Leader D was the most assertive email I've ever sent in my life. I was, though perhaps Leader D and others at Large Nonprofit Health System would disagree, still respectful. But I didn't hold anything back. I let them know what was happening from my perspective, and I begged for their help in getting people to take what I was sharing seriously and allow me to remain at the table.

The collaborative, deferential approach I'd been trying wasn't working. I was losing the fight, and I knew it.

My change in tone came about when I realized that I had very few options left. I could keep playing it safe, trying time after time to respectfully collaborate with people who had zero intention of collaborating with me. Or I could step outside of my comfort zone and lay it all out there, putting my heart on the line, with the hope that maybe, just maybe, it would get someone to have a real conversation with me.

CHAPTER 14

Day 435 and a Half

Learning About Bridget

Twelve hours later. Over 430 days from when I'd first sounded the alarm that we had holes to address and mothers at risk. 12:30 a.m.

I'd sent the boldest email of my entire life more than 12 hours ago, and I hadn't heard anything back. Not an "I'm so sorry, let's talk about this ASAP," and not even an "Emily, this message was highly inappropriate. I'd like to talk ASAP, and you might want to start packing your things."

Just even more deafening silence.

I was dumbfounded, and I was beginning to panic. Frustrated as I was, I'd still been clinging to the hope that somehow, in some way, I would be able to get people to see what I was seeing, and we would get to work on closing the important gaps in care that I'd so diligently reported to my leaders over a year prior.

What is going on?

I've been trained on how to recognize process failures and how to resolve them.

I've consistently gotten strong feedback from the leaders I work with.

Now, I'm coming to them with an opportunity to not only improve the way we care for new moms but to publicly demonstrate our commitment to quality improvement and patient safety.

These are good people. I'm a good person. I know that they know that I'm a good person.

I've been nothing but consistent in the way I show up in the workplace and in explaining what my motives and objectives are.

WHAT THE HELL IS GOING ON?!

This was a question that haunted me (and sometimes still does). I generally pride myself on being able to see multiple sides of an issue, regardless of where I stand personally. But not with this situation: I could not concoct a plausible reason why healthcare leaders who knew me and knew my capabilities would be shutting me out of the conversation on this topic.[xix]

It has to be a legal issue.

But I'm not a threat. I have no lasting damage (physically) from my experience, and I've said and shown repeatedly that I wish to be fully transparent and that my goal is to improve our system.

So, once again… WHAT IS GOING ON?

And then an idea popped into my head.

---

xix   For anyone thinking, "Honey, of course any reasonable organization would stop talking to you out of liability concerns," I'll address that in Part 3. That's not currently an evidence-based opinion for the healthcare industry.

I wonder if…

I pulled up ChatGPT, which I'd just recently learned how to use as part of my research and advocacy work. I instructed it to "scan local obituaries and see if you can find any women who have died in the last year in [my state] with references to postpartum depression or suicide."

Half a second later, ChatGPT responded, and my heart sank. There she was.

Bridget: a mother of three, including a three-month old. An obituary requesting donations to suicide-prevention organizations.

"Wait a minute… this can't be real. What if…" I thought, as I frantically looked her up on social media.

Her profile was public, and there it was. Photos of her in the hospital after giving birth to her youngest child. I thought I recognized the background and the furniture in the hospital room, but I didn't want to jump to conclusions too fast. So, I looked up photo galleries of local birth centers to confirm what I already knew: Bridget had given birth at one of Large Nonprofit Health System's hospitals.

My heart was pounding. Tears were streaming down my face.

"No, this isn't supposed to keep happening," I said out loud, in the middle of the night, to nobody.

I learned that Bridget had died the preceding May. *Nearly six months (Day 153, to be exact) after* I'd started sounding the alarm about gaping holes in our care processes that made this kind of result possible. Three months after I'd backed off after sensing a painful wall of indifference that I couldn't yet face.

A wave of guilt washed over me.

What if I hadn't given up on those conversations with Leader A? What if I'd been more adamant that we make changes? Would this have happened? Would those three kids still have a mom?

As I do in times of crisis, I called my own mom.

Though it was the middle of the night, she picked up, and I shared what I'd just learned.

"Oh, sweetie…," she replied. "I am so sorry. I am so, so sorry." Worst of all, though my mom was surprised to get a call from me at that hour, she wasn't particularly surprised at the news I was sharing. Like me, she had firsthand experience of the gaps in care and knowledge related to maternal mental health; like me, she'd been grasping at straws to understand the response I'd been getting when trying to advocate for changes to be made.

———

That night, I made myself a promise.

You did what you could. You shared what you knew, and you shared how to begin moving forward. It's not your fault that they didn't listen, and it's not your fault that you couldn't continue spearheading this conversation under the suffocating weight of indifference.

But…

It sure as hell means I need a new approach. Never again will I allow someone to gaslight me into thinking that the gaps I see don't exist, or that this issue is anything but urgent.

Fool me once, shame on you. Fool me twice, shame on me.

Maternal Mental Health Has No Political Party

There's one more thing that's important to note about Bridget and the impact her story has had on my advocacy journey.

Bridget was also a white woman. Aside from that, from what I can tell, we actually had very little in common.

Bridget was a deeply religious stay-at-home mom. I've never been to a single church service in my entire life, and I'm a happily working mother. Bridget was anti-vax; I'm married to a doctor and wouldn't dream of skipping or delaying a single vaccine for my son. And the list of our differences goes on.

But postpartum mental health disorders don't care who you voted for. They can impact anyone.

If anything, learning that Bridget and I were so ideologically opposed gave me the energy to fight this fight even harder. It showed me that this issue transcends the divisions tearing our country apart. Supporting the mental health of new mothers might just be one thing we can all agree on. And solving a crisis this big will require all of us: Democrats, Republicans, and everyone in between.

Disclaimer: I don't know the details of Bridget's story. All I know is what I saw on social media, her obituary, and her family's GoFundMe. I don't know if she did, or didn't, seek help from her healthcare team during her struggle with postpartum anxiety and depression, or even who her primary healthcare team was. But I *am* reasonably certain that she gave birth at one of Large Nonprofit Health System's hospitals, and that Large Nonprofit Health System could've done more to prevent an outcome like hers, because many of the suggestions

I'd offered (including but not limited to educating all of our perinatal providers about the signs, symptoms, and risk factors for maternal mental health disorders) were still waiting in "competing priorities" purgatory.

CHAPTER 15

Day 436

A New Advocacy Chapter Begins

Learning about Bridget fundamentally changed me.

I'd already ratcheted up my intensity level and lost much of my filter (at least from behind the wall of a computer screen), as demonstrated by my email to Leader D.

But this was different.

Learning about and digesting the news of Bridget's death taught me to trust my training, my experience, and my intuition like never before. It taught me that people in positions of authority can make mistakes, and that inaction by those in power can cause irreparable harm.

The next morning, I got a response from Leader D.

They apologized, but in an "I'm sorry you feel that way" kind of way, complete with boilerplate language around Large Nonprofit Health System's commitment to patient feedback and continual improvement and an insinuation that they would continue the work without me.

Once again, they were putting me in the patient "box," patting themselves on the back for work already underway, and (in my opinion) implying that the biggest problem at hand was my level of patience.

But the most painful thing of all was that the tone of this email was an abrupt change from any other interaction I'd ever had with Leader D.

We'd had one-on-one conversations about sensitive subjects such as the role of gender in the workplace and the impact of racism and structural inequities on healthcare access and outcomes. I'd deeply admired their willingness to face challenging issues head-on, as well as their eagerness to use their experience and wisdom to support, encourage, and mentor the next generation of healthcare leaders.

So, when this email came through, I pictured them either writing that message with someone from the Large Nonprofit Health System legal team standing *directly* over their shoulder or perhaps asking AI to draft the most generic, distant, and deflective response possible to the email I'd sent.

Anything to avoid needing to rewrite the narrative in my head about the leader I thought, and hoped, they were.

Preparing for Battle

I had a weekend between the discovery of Bridget's obituary (and the response from Leader D) and the meeting with Leader A and Leader B. Deb had at some point been cut loose from this conversation.

I spent much of that weekend preparing, so that I could make the most of the short time we had and to demonstrate that I came armed with research and ready to collaborate and move forward.

By the time Monday rolled around, I was ready. I'd spent hundreds of dollars printing out carefully curated articles and reports, and I'd put together a concise, two-page vision of how we could move forward with all of the information at hand.

I put on a blazer over my Large Nonprofit Health System T-shirt, added my lucky bracelet, and headed into the office.

The first thing Leader A said to me after we sat down was something to the effect of "I know we don't have much time on the calendar today, so I wanted to clarify the purpose of our conversation and what we hope to get out of it. We're here to hear more about *your experience as a patient* with our care system, and how we could have done better *in your case*."

I paused. The room was silent for a moment.

Once again, I could feel them desperately trying to put me in a box: to separate my lived experience from my professional expertise.

"That's interesting," I said. "Because that's not why I'm here. We've already talked quite a bit about my personal experience, which I'm grateful for. I'm here to share my thoughts as a leader at Large Nonprofit Health System on how we should move forward on this issue, and to request a seat at the table as we do."

They smiled gently, though with a touch of sadness, and gave me a quick nod.

In that short meeting, I did my best to lay out everything I knew about the problem, all of the current resources and research, and how I'd suggest moving forward in light of all of it. I was transparent, prepared, and clear. At times, I was emotional. Not overly so, in my opinion; simply on par with the emotional weight of the work I was attempting to champion.

I shared it all: why I'd taken a step back a year prior after receiving an email that felt like a subtle "go away," and why I'd resumed my efforts after I met the CEO of Other Local Health System and heard that the PHP in our area struggled with utilization. I even shared what I'd found when I went looking in the middle of the night for explanations to the decidedly cold shoulder I'd been getting: Bridget's obituary.

I pleaded with them to allow me in, to embrace my story and the insights it offered rather than push me away.

I reminded them that the prevailing philosophy on patient safety within healthcare administration is that feedback should be embraced, not buried, and that we should be focusing on bolstering our processes rather than blaming any of our providers individually.

The meeting was civil, and it ended politely.

As I always do, I thanked them for their time and their willingness to hear my perspective. And I went back down to my desk, hoping for a miracle yet knowing it was unlikely.

Go Away; Goodbye

Just a few hours later, I got a follow-up message from Leader A.

It was short. They thanked me for the meeting, and for the research, resources, and experiences I'd offered, and they assured me that all of it would inform *their* perinatal mental health improvement work—without me.

That was it.

After hours of research, hours of preparation, and an impassioned plea to volunteer my time and expertise to improve our system and lead the way for others, I received a less than 100-word response essentially saying, yet again, "Thanks, but no thanks."

CHAPTER 16

Day 440

Women Are Dying, Deb

After taking a few days to "cool down" after this disappointing message, I had a realization: this was just one person's opinion. An extremely important person, given their role in the organization, but still just one person. There was too much on the line, too many women's and babies' lives in the balance, for me to give up based on resistance from a single individual. After all, most other people I spoke to about my experience, including Leader C (originally, at least), had a very different reaction: one of horror, gratitude for the information, and an instinct to act.

So, once again, I put my head down, gave my best to the other projects I was working on that were completely unrelated to maternal health, and continued to strategize about how to move forward. I shifted my advocacy focus to the upcoming conference, where I was going to share my story with hundreds of people.

Given the response from my leadership team, I had to revise the end of my speech, because it was clear that I could no longer conclude with any sincere statements about actions my own organization had taken, or even vowed to take, in light of my story.

One day, I made a comment to Deb about the upcoming conference. When I'd first mentioned the speaking opportunity to them a month prior, they'd seemed supportive and excited for me. What they said next therefore confused me: "When you're finished drafting your speech, you might want to consider running it by our communications team."

I paused, unsure what to make of that suggestion.

I thought maybe a clarification would help: "Well, I've asked several times if Large Nonprofit Health System might be willing to sponsor the conference so that I can attend in part as a representative of the organization. I thought the answer was that I need to do this entirely as an individual, on my own time, with my own resources."

I paused to see if that was their understanding as well. It was.

"So, if I'm going entirely as an individual, not associated with Large Nonprofit Health System in any way, why would I run my speech by our communications team? I don't understand."

Deb seemed flustered.

"Well, I'm just saying, you're always an employee," they responded. "You just might want to be careful, that's all."

Anger started rising within me. I was almost finished with the second draft of my speech, and as with anything I do or say, it was honest but respectful. I hadn't named names, and I'd focused on patterns that I know to be true across the country, not just within my own organization.

I wasn't actually concerned that our communications team would want to change much, if anything, about what I'd written. But the mere suggestion that I should run my content by our communications team, for the possibility of censorship without any offer of backing or support, was pretty damn insulting.

Why would they want to censor me?

Yes, I know the answer seems obvious. They might not have wanted me to share the healthcare "misses" I'd experienced and the underlying gaps they revealed, because they weren't yet comfortable acknowledging or owning the very real fact that those gaps, indeed, existed.

But to me, at that time, it was confusing. I'd been part of this organization for several years, working closely with senior leaders the entire time. I was proud of the work we did and of what I thought was evidence of a forward-thinking, mission-oriented organization that deeply valued its people and, at the center of it all, its patients.

That single conversation with Deb was the one that finally shattered the illusion for me. Even more so than the short email I'd received from Leader A dismissing the hours upon hours of free expertise and labor I'd offered, this conversation with Deb illuminated something I'd been avoiding at all costs.

This exchange made me feel like maybe, just maybe, there was something equally or *more* important to the leaders of my organization than eliminating preventable harm: upholding Large Nonprofit Health System's reputation. Specifically, upholding the self-selected reputation of being patient-centered and deeply committed to quality improvement, while somehow never admitting to process gaps that might actually warrant improvement or allowing the voice of a patient to be a part of the improvement process.

If it hadn't been for my recent discovery of Bridget's story, it's possible that I might have caved and worked with the communications team to ensure that all boxes had been checked and not a single soul would be mad at me for what I shared with the world next.[xx]

But like I said, learning about Bridget fundamentally changed me. I now realized that I held important experience and expertise that the world needed to hear, and that the systems that were holding me back from making change were the same ones that were continuing to allow harm to come to others: others like Bridget and, by extension, her children.

I teared up in this conversation with Deb.[xxi]

I stood my ground, and I simply responded, "Women are dying, Deb. There are kids who are growing up without their parents who don't need to be. I need to be honest about what happened."

They nodded, and then they backed off.

The Maternal Mental Health Forum

I like to think that I found a chink in the armor in that conversation, and that Deb had seen the stakes from my perspective, because they were nothing but supportive from then on.

Fast-forward a month or so, and I took almost an entire week of PTO to fly out to Washington, D.C. to publicly share my story out loud for the first time at the Maternal Mental Health Forum, hosted by the Policy Center for Maternal Mental Health. I flew alone with my toddler in my lap so we could visit a friend before the conference. As someone whose parenthood journey had started with a near-deadly level of anxiety, this alone felt like a monumental accomplishment.

---

xx   Because, as for many other recovering "pleasure to have in class" sort of kids, people not liking me has basically equated to "DANGER!!! THREAT LEVEL MIDNIGHT!" in my brain for most of my life.

xxi   I have come to learn and appreciate that showing emotion in the workplace, especially if you work in healthcare, is not a sign of weakness or the inability to think clearly or rationally. On the contrary, it's often a sign that you recognize the weight of the work and the impact of your actions (or inactions) on the lives of other human beings.

My mom and my aunt eventually met us out there and came to the conference with me.

My experience at the conference was redemptive. After months and months of people looking the other way and giving me the cold shoulder when I spoke up about this topic, I was now in a room surrounded by hundreds of other people who were fighting in some way to change the narrative for new parents. Many of them were healthcare leaders themselves. People cried, people thanked me for my honesty, people acknowledged that much of what I'd been through was avoidable and shouldn't have ever happened.

The conference showed me, definitively, that the problem lay not with me but with an organization that wasn't ready or willing to accept their role in the problem or the solution.

CHAPTER 17

Day 480

Once I was back at work and the conference recordings were posted online, I sent a note to Leader C.

In this note, I provided the link to my short speech and shared with them that I'd been feeling "pegged" as a liability: the very thing we'd discussed trying to avoid in our first meeting.

The response was, as you've probably come to expect, discouraging. They validated that I wasn't a liability, but they took what I interpreted as a subtle jab at my patience.

Sigh. In retrospect, it all feels a bit like my toddler, who always wants to have the last word. Or when I ask him to please stop putting food in his milk and he yells back, "Be NICE, Mama! Be NICE."

While Large Nonprofit Health System leaders never stated this quite so explicitly, along the way, I often felt like I was being told, "Thank you; you're helping us improve. BUT… I just want to remind you again that your unreasonable expectations are also a problem."

If there's any chance you're siding with Leader C on this one right now, I'd like to gently remind you that we were almost 500 days out from my initial feedback, and I had yet to see or hear about *a single change* being made in light of it.

While the conversation remained civil, as always, it ended abruptly, as we agreed to discuss the matter in person.

You're Too Close

I dropped by their office one day the following week when I noticed that their computer "dot" was green and their calendar appeared open.

"Oh, hi Emily, come on in," they said when they heard me gently knock on the door.

But the tone of the conversation quickly turned cold: a stark contrast to all the other in-person interactions I'd ever had with them.

I thanked them for the offer to talk about our last conversation (always lead with gratitude!), and I asked for further clarification.

They asked me, "You keep stressing the need to involve lived experience, but you've offered your feedback, and the team has received it. What more are you looking for?"

I was dumbfounded.

This person was in one of the highest levels of healthcare leadership, but they were genuinely asking me what could be missing in this equation. I tried to kindly, but clearly, explain the gap.

"I appreciate that I've had the chance to share my feedback. But I keep hearing that maternal mental health has been adequately addressed because of one change that's been made, unrelated to the feedback that I've shared.[xxii] But the *whole point* of what I've shared is that transforming maternal mental healthcare isn't as simple as implementing one or two new process improvements or solutions. The point is that *the entire care journey* needs an honest, thorough review, guided by people who've been impacted by it."

---

xxii   A change that, genuinely, was a great one.

Another way to think about it: why did it make sense for me to wait until the team had finished their work in a silo, then see the output and inevitably have feedback about what they'd missed, rather than join the team now so I could help them see and address gaps as they worked?

Furthermore, given what I'd learned along the way about how we used to, not very long ago, *routinely implement depression screenings for new moms and then literally do *nothing* even when they self-disclosed thoughts of self-harm or suicide*, I had reservations about whether a team of individuals without lived experience would be able to fully transform the process.

To make matters worse, Large Nonprofit Health System was, like so many health systems, proud of meeting that universal screening checkbox. But in my opinion, they, along with all other health systems who universally screen patients but don't have a clear, consistent, and robust follow-up plan, lacked the humility to acknowledge that screening without adequate follow-up action isn't helpful; it can actually be quite harmful.

I don't remember everything Leader C said in this conversation, but I do remember them uttering the words, "You can't just invite yourself to the table, Emily" and "You're too close."

They went on to tell me that the team had asked for "space" [presumably from me], and that they were inclined to give it to them.

I quickly gathered that the days of this senior leader validating my experiences and my leadership potential were behind us, and that I needed to find a way to exit the room and the conversation before I exploded in anger and devastation about the harm that would inevitably continue to come to new moms and babies in the absence of true reform.

At one point before I left, they asked, "Would it help if you could get an update of some kind on the work that they're doing, so you can see that things are moving forward? I can check in with Leader A and let them know you would find that meaningful."

"Yes, I would really appreciate that," I replied.

I once again thanked them profusely for their time and their willingness to hear my opinion, then exited the room, knowing that it was all over. The case was closed.

To add insult to injury, that update from Leader A never came.

CHAPTER 18

Day 515

Walking Away

One month later, over 500 days from when I'd first spoken up about my experience, I handed in my resignation notice. It was incredibly bittersweet.

I loved my job, and I was deeply entrenched in multiple projects that I was proud to be a part of. At home, my husband and I were independently financially comfortable for the very first time in our adult lives.

Quitting my job meant abandoning those projects, leaving behind a deep internal network that I'd worked hard to build and maintain, transitioning from a respectable mid-level salary to a part-time youth sports coach salary, and walking straight into the unknown.

But to be honest, after that last conversation with Leader C, I never really felt like I had a choice. Thankfully, my husband agreed.

From that point on, I felt that I wasn't welcome in conversations about improving maternal mental health at Large Nonprofit Health System. But given what I'd already learned about the state of maternal mental health in America, *not* taking any part in maternal mental health improvement was not an option to me. And if I couldn't somehow tie that work to my day job, I simply didn't have enough hours in the day to do it all. By this point, I had more conferences and speaking engagements already on the calendar and people in the field whom I wanted to connect with, and I didn't have enough time to squeeze that in between Julian's bedtime and mine.

That's the nice way to put it.

The less-nice way to put it was that this experience was a sobering reality check for me: I realized that Large Nonprofit Health System, in my opinion, was less committed to the mission and ideals that I'd signed up for than I'd once thought. My experience with maternal mental health led me to question everything else I was working toward but facing barriers to. Was it difficult to get things done because that's just life, and things take a while? Or was it difficult to get things done because, at the end of the day, what the organization said it was about and what it was *actually* about were two separate things?

As a healthcare administrator, I didn't want to work for leaders whose interpretation of "centering lived experience" meant taking a point-in-time piece of feedback and running (away) with it. I didn't want to work for an organization that talked about the need to reduce mental health stigma while simultaneously perpetuating structures and processes that inherently stigmatized mental health.

While I loved my job, in terms of both its day-to-day content and the stability and security it provided my family, I knew it was time to walk away.

Thank You, Deb

Not everyone has the ability to make that decision, and I recognize that.

If anything, it was another reason I felt that I *needed* to walk away. Because if I, someone with immense amounts of privilege (including the ability to patch things together financially for a couple years until my husband finished residency), wouldn't stand my ground on this, who would?

The time had come for me to put my money where my mouth was (literally), and I did.

On the day I turned in my notice, I cried.

I think, though my memory of this interaction is fuzzy, and it's possible I'm simply imagining it, Deb also cried.

They told me they were sad about my decision, but that they understood and, most importantly, respected it. They gave me a hug, wished me luck, and validated that I'd repeatedly "taken the high road" and that they understood my need to leave.

I told them how much their leadership meant to me, and I meant every word of it.

Deb was a phenomenal leader in many ways, but the factor that's most relevant here is the way in which they had the humility to change their tune when presented with new information.

I'd been horrified at their suggestion that I work with an internal team to presumably censor some of my writing, despite writing and presenting strictly as an individual. I challenged that suggestion with a clear reason, and they backed off. From then on, they were vehemently supportive of every step in my advocacy journey.

I'm coming to learn that humility is perhaps the most important quality in a healthcare leader or organization. It's difficult to improve anything if you can't also acknowledge that things aren't as good as they could be. And as long as people try to hold on to recognition and praise for improvement and growth without ever actually admitting to the shortcomings that create an opportunity for improvement in the first place, we won't make any significant progress.

To truly move forward, sometimes we need to be able to accept that maybe we were wrong.

As a leader, that means the willingness to accept that maybe you've made a bad call at some point. As an organization, that means the willingness to talk about the gaps you've identified that eventually led to improvements, not just harping on the improvements themselves as if it's possible to improve upon things that are already perfect.

Moving forward with maternal mental health in the U.S., as with many other topics, is going to require quite a bit of humility.

It will require health systems to acknowledge that, perhaps, we lack the infrastructure needed to adequately support new moms and, by extension, their babies (we do).

It will require payers to acknowledge that this gap exists, in part, because maternal mental healthcare hasn't been adequately compensated (it hasn't).

It will require policymakers to acknowledge that our lack of paid leave and other societal-level support for new parents leaves our population *much* more vulnerable to maternal mental health disorders (it does).

If you're reading this, Deb, thank you for giving me the confidence that somebody in healthcare leadership cared about what happened to me: enough to want to prevent it from happening to others.

PART 3

The Bigger Picture—Gaps in the U.S. Healthcare Infrastructure

Worth More Dead Than Alive? How Fear of Liability (Still) Keeps Healthcare From Hearing the Harmed

I refuse to believe that the leaders at Large Nonprofit Health System don't value the lives of women and their babies. I also doubt that they suddenly questioned my competence or leadership ability.

In light of those beliefs, the only plausible reason, in my opinion, that I was kept out of conversations about maternal mental health was a concern about liability.

But here's the thing: the approach of barring those with bad experiences from the room is not currently an evidence-based healthcare leadership strategy.

As I mentioned earlier, I'm a relatively recent graduate of a highly respected MHA program. Here are a few of the things I learned in that program:

- Most issues in healthcare are rooted in systems failures. If we want to solve big problems, we have to design

- strong systems: ones that leave less room for accidents or oversights that lead to patient harm.
- Leaders shouldn't fear feedback; they should seek it. Feedback about misses, as well as near misses and even inconsequential mistakes, is the critical information we need to build stronger systems.
- When healthcare errors result in harm, apologizing and making a good faith effort to correct the issue actually reduces, rather than increases, liability.

I know that last bullet point is counterintuitive to many, including my traditional businessman father, whom I mentioned earlier. His immediate reaction to my predicament with Large Nonprofit Health System was, "Of course they don't want to admit that there are any gaps, because then they would be admitting to wrongdoing and opening themselves up to liability!"

But the reverse is true, and anyone who's been harmed by healthcare can probably understand the mechanism behind this. People want to know that their experiences matter and that by speaking up, they can prevent similar harm from coming to others. Lawsuits can be time-consuming and traumatizing; more often than not, what patients are really after is accountability.

I was happy to correct my dad and tell him that "admitting responsibility increases liability" is a myth. It's been disproven by multiple studies showing that transparency, apology, and proactive improvements *reduce* both the number of lawsuits and litigation costs.[24]

In 2016, the federal Agency for Healthcare Research and Quality (AHRQ) introduced the Communication and Optimal Resolution (CANDOR) toolkit to help hospitals change their approach to handling patient harm and malpractice suits, based in part on earlier successes at places like Michigan Medicine. The toolkit was intended to help address the "invisible wall of silence—built out of legal worries" that often leaves families in the dark and "keeps doctors, nurses, and others from being able to learn from mistakes and near-misses."[25]

In place of silence, the CANDOR toolkit emphasizes the value in removing barriers to reporting harms, errors, and near misses, using this information for process improvement, and engaging in proactive and transparent communication. The stated goal is to "improve safety, serve patients better, reduce the emotional toll on clinicians and resolve situations fairly—with litigation as a last resort."[26]

I can't be certain, but I'd venture a guess that the problem at Large Nonprofit Health System was *not* lack of awareness of this framework. I'm pretty confident that Large Nonprofit Health System leaders, and especially risk management leaders, stay apprised of the latest research and are aware of CANDOR. In fact, if you had a meet and greet with our risk management team (like I could have had, in theory, when I was an administrative fellow), I bet they'd even spout all of this exact ideology to you.

But unfortunately, nearly a decade after the release of the CANDOR toolkit, my experience suggests that perhaps some health systems are doing a better job of *talking* about best practices in liability and patient safety than actually *implementing* them.

Swiss Cheese

The "Swiss cheese model" is a commonly used phrase in health-care. It means that if you combine multiple safety measures, you reduce the risk of harm by eliminating situations where a single process failure leads to significant harm. Human error, for example, is a fact of life, but by combining multiple safety measures, you can reduce the risk of human error leading to patient harm. It's a way of building stronger systems. It's also a way of shifting blame away from individual providers when something goes awry, because blaming and shaming individual providers for mistakes that could have been prevented through stronger systems is not a good use of anyone's time.

I believe in this model so deeply that I use it in my own home and demand that my son's other frequent caretakers do the same. When it comes to preventing accidents, we don't rely on just one layer of protection. For example, we keep a close eye on Julian if he's in the kitchen, *and* we have stove burner covers to prevent him from accidentally turning the gas stove on. The door to the bathroom stays closed, *and* there are child locks on the bathroom cabinet that contains cleaning supplies.

This way, if one of us is having an off day and forgets to close the door to the bathroom, there's another layer of safety between my son and him consuming Windex. This isn't rocket science, just common-sense risk reduction through layered protections. I'm adamant about using this model in my home, because while I know that I can't control everything, I know that I can control some things, and those things can meaningfully decrease my son's risk of accidental injury (the leading cause of child death in the United States).[27]

The same thing often applies in healthcare. No matter how hard we try or how much we invest in patient safety efforts, we can't control everything. There will be accidents, human errors, unforeseen circumstances, unique patient presentations, and so on. But there are some things that *are* in our control, including how many layers of protection we stack between our patients and harm's way. In healthcare, these "layers" might include checklists, electronic alerts, staff training, and backup protocols, all designed to catch what one individual might miss.

But how do you identify the potential gaps, or the layers of protection that would help prevent harm? After all, we're talking about healthcare processes now, not easily visible holes in a piece of cheese that anybody can see.

The fastest way to do this is to ask the people who've been through that healthcare process, and particularly those who didn't have the intended outcome. *Those* are the people who know where the holes are, because those are the people who fell through them.

Any attempt to improve complex systems without involving the people who've had personal experiences with those systems will inevitably fall short. Not because of lack of intelligence or lack of effort, but because it can sometimes be impossible to see things you haven't personally experienced.

Seeking Information

Though I didn't personally *need* an experiential learning experience to take these patient safety and risk mitigation lessons to heart, my own experiences following my postpartum mental health crisis drove the rationale behind these lessons home.

Bringing a lawsuit against Large Nonprofit Health System for the several, clearly documented ways in which they dropped the ball during my mental health crisis did not cross my mind, even once, for nearly two years.

I am privileged, in so many ways. For starters, I was lucky enough to survive, and that alone is reason for me to care more about paying it forward by addressing gaps in care than seeking personal remuneration. Secondly, while we aren't rolling in money, we aren't buried under medical debt, either. So, I didn't need to pursue legal action in order to pay my bills or make ends meet.

The first time I came up against a wall in my internal advocacy efforts, I figured it was my fault: I wasn't ready yet, I didn't have all of my research together, I hadn't made a strong enough case. But a year later, when I came up against that same wall despite now having all of my ducks in a row, I realized there might be something bigger going on, something more ominous.

I felt unseen, disrespected, angry. Above all, I felt *desperate* for a way to get the Large Nonprofit Health System leaders' attention and to ensure that addressing the gaps in care was not considered optional. One day, while I was talking to a friend, she asked if I'd considered bringing a lawsuit against Large Nonprofit Health System.

"No." I was adamant. "I'm not doing that. Litigation isn't the best way of solving problems in healthcare."

"Okay, but just think about it," she responded. "I think you have a strong case. And that'll get their attention."

This sat in the back of my mind for a few days.

Wait, could I really sue them for what happened? My experiences with the health system directly contributed to my suicidality, which took me down a financially costly and emotionally excruciating journey...

But litigation is the exact opposite of how I learned to problem-solve in healthcare.

But it might be the only way of getting them to pay attention to me. If I sue them and win, maybe they'll have no choice but to address the process gaps I've raised. But, but, but...

I was torn.

I opted to get in contact with a few lawyers, just to understand what my options were; regardless of what they said, I might as well get that information (after all, as I hope you're noticing, I aspire to always take a "let's not fear information" stance).[xxiii]

I reached out to someone in my network and got recommendations for reputable medical malpractice lawyers in my area. I pored through my medical notes in more detail than I'd done before, documenting dates and times and responses and actions and inactions. I prepared a summary, and I made a few calls.

In summary, what I learned by talking with a few lawyers was that emotional damage alone is rarely enough to entice lawyers to take your case. Cases involving permanent damage and loss are more compelling, given the inherent costs associated with litigation.

These conversations were tough, because hearing that you have to die or sustain permanent damage for people to *really* care about what happened to you is a tough pill to swallow.

Reflecting on those conversations and how they made me feel brought me back to my original stance: litigation was not the best way forward. It wouldn't be the best use of my time and resources, and it wouldn't be the best use of Large Nonprofit Health System's time and resources, either. And in the end, all I've ever wanted was to ensure that no other family had to suffer and struggle the way mine did.

This sentiment is true of many survivors of adverse events and patient harm, and it's at the very heart of the CANDOR toolkit and current wisdom on patient safety philosophy.

---

xxiii This is something I ultimately shared with Large Nonprofit Health System leaders, in the name of complete transparency.

The Cost of Being Alive

My mom is a fighter. She's smart, she does her research, and she advocates *fiercely* for her children.

A scenario played out in my head: one in which I'd died and my mom had channeled her grief into action, and had sued Large Nonprofit Health System. I pictured her winning. I pictured her being outspoken and talking to the media about it. I pictured her doing every damn thing in her power to ensure no other family would have to endure the pain that she did.

After all, the essay I'd written and published aimed at Large Nonprofit Health System (the hypothetical one where the leaders who'd known me personally took a heroic sequence of steps, resulting in stronger infrastructure for families in our area) was always the best-case hypothetical scenario.

But I'd always known that they also could've taken the "deny and defend" approach, after which my family might have come after them with legal action. I pictured this happening, and the good that might've come out of this issue being thrust into the light by grieving parents unwilling to settle for anything less than substantial change, especially if they won that case.

I tried explaining this to people in my family: that the message I was receiving through this brief legal exploration process was that *in terms of bringing change to the healthcare system*, perhaps I would've been worth more dead than alive. But given my now-history with depression, people predictably started getting a little antsy. "No, don't say that. That's not true."

In general, I'm worth so much more alive. I know this. Particularly to Julian, who matters more to me than any career or crusade. So, I want to clarify, in case anyone still feels skittish:

if I had to choose between transforming healthcare or being alive to mother my son, I'd choose my son, every single time.

But I'm going to make my family uncomfortable yet again and maintain my original stance: my experience of talking to lawyers told me that in terms of getting the attention of local healthcare leaders, **I may have been worth more dead than alive.**

As I say, regardless of the implicit message I received through that process, I know the opposite is true. I'm worth way more alive. Not just to my family and friends but to the healthcare world, too. I know that I have the insight, the tools, the knowledge, the connections, and the fire to drive change. I know that, eventually, this will become clear to everyone, including the leaders at Large Nonprofit Health System.

I just wish I hadn't had to walk away from my hard-earned career and share my personal trauma in vivid detail for the whole world to see in order to prove that.

CHAPTER 20

An Aside on American Culture

Before I talk any more about gaps in maternal mental healthcare, I should first acknowledge that part of the problem with maternal mental health in the United States isn't medical at all. It's cultural.

While other countries protect and honor new mothers with rituals that include rest, relaxation, and nurturing from others, the United States does not. Here, most people go it alone during the newborn stage, independently responsible for the 24/7 task of sustaining a new human life just a few days after childbirth or major abdominal surgery.

Paid maternity leave is scarce;[28] paid paternity or parental leave for partners is even scarcer. Those who dare to openly question this reality are often quietly (or not so quietly) viewed as lazy, ungrateful, impractical, or simply not up to the monumental task of being a parent.

I recognize that considering all maternal mental health disorders as pathological conditions requiring medical treatment is a distinctly Western view. I also recognize that, in reality, we could probably make just as much improvement in this area by radically transforming our cultural traditions surrounding childbirth and the postpartum period.

However, just as we could similarly improve diabetes and obesity care by radically transforming our food and exercise habits in America, we generally choose to invest in the medical facilities and medications needed to treat the known health repercussions of those conditions. Doctors are trained in how to treat medical conditions, regardless of whether societal changes could reduce their frequency.

So, for the purpose of this book, I'm focusing on healthcare-oriented solutions to a problem that we know exists and can be effectively treated by healthcare professionals. But before I move on, I want to acknowledge some of the customs and rituals from other countries that undoubtedly have a positive impact on the mental health of new parents. A UK-based organization called The Mindful Birth Group summarized this well in their blog post titled "Postnatal Rituals From Around The World,"[29] which I have shared below with their permission.

Postnatal Rituals From Around The World
Author: The Mindful Birth Group

South Korea: New mums/parents traditionally observe a 21-day confinement period called sanhujori, during which they avoid going outside and receiving guests. The new mum/parent is cared for by their mother or mother-in-law, who prepares special foods and supports with breastfeeding.

Mexico: New mums/parents are cared for by a traditional midwife or partera during the postnatal period. The midwife provides massages and herbal remedies to help with recovery and healing.

India: New mums/parents observe a 40-day confinement period called jaapa, during which they rest and are cared for by family members. The mother/parent is fed special foods and drinks, and a special massage is performed using warm herbal oils.

China: New mums/parents observe a confinement period called zuò yuè zi, during which they avoid leaving the house and receive daily massages from a traditional practitioner. The new mum/parent is also given special foods and drinks to promote healing and lactation.

Morocco: New mums/parents observe a 40-day confinement period called al-taqsan, during which they are cared for by their mother or mother-in-law. The new mum/parent is given special foods and drinks to promote healing and lactation, and daily massages are performed to help with recovery.

Iceland: New mums/parents observe a tradition called rúntur, during which they take a walk around their town or village with their newborn to introduce the baby to the community. This tradition is believed to bring good luck and support to the new family.

Japan: New mums/parents observe a 100-day confinement period called osouji, during which they avoid leaving the house and are cared for by their mother or mother-in-law. The new mum/parent is given special foods and drinks, and a special massage is performed to help with recovery.

Brazil: New mums/parents are encouraged to take a 40-day break from their regular activities after childbirth, known as resguardo. During this time, new mums/parents avoid going outside and are cared for by family members. Special foods and drinks are prepared to promote healing and lactation.

Nigeria: New mums/parents observe a 30-day confinement period called omugwo, during which they are cared for by their mother or mother-in-law. The new mum/parent is given special foods and drinks, and daily massages are performed to help with recovery.

Australia: In some Indigenous Australian cultures, new mums/parents observe a traditional practice called yarning circles, during which they gather with other mums/parents to share their experiences and receive support during the postnatal period.

Do you see a pattern here?

Other countries recognize childbirth as the physically, mentally, and emotionally taxing event that it is: one that warrants an explicit period of rest and healing.

But here in the U.S., most mothers are often on their own shortly after hospital discharge, taking care of themselves, a newborn baby, household chores, and perhaps other children and animals. And to make it worse, this period of maternity leave (if you're lucky enough to get enough time away from work to call it that) is sometimes referred to by male and/or childless colleagues as "vacation."

CHAPTER 21

The Doctors Know Less Than You Think

They Won't Know If We Don't Teach Them

Maternal mental health is not routinely covered in U.S. medical education.

Not in medical school, and not in residency programs, even for specialties such as OBGYN, family medicine, pediatrics, or psychiatry, which routinely care for and/or interact with pregnant and postpartum women.

My husband is a fairly recent graduate of a well-respected medical school, and maternal mental health was not a subject that they covered; nor has it been covered in his internal medicine residency thus far. And no, a passing slide or two on "the baby blues" vs. "postpartum depression" doesn't count.

I've also, more often than you'd think, gotten responses to my tales of nightmarish doctor appointments such as, "Oh, I can relate. I told my OB that I hadn't slept in days, and she suggested I try drinking tea." OBGYNs and perinatal psychiatrists have also told me directly that everything they've learned on this topic has been self-directed.

But my evidence of this training gap isn't strictly anecdotal. In 2015, which is just one decade ago at the time of writing, a study was published in the *American Journal of Psychiatry* where the researchers had surveyed residency directors. They found that only 59% of psychiatry residency programs required any level of training in reproductive psychiatry, and that only 36% of respondents believed all residents need to be competent in the field.[30]

Stop and think about that for a moment. Women make up 50% of the population, and more than 85% of women will give birth at some point in their lives.[31] Yet more than a third of psychiatric training program leaders didn't think their residents needed basic competence in perinatal mental health.

How could that be?

Well, for one, the people making decisions about medical curricula are predominantly men, who've never personally navigated pregnancy, birth, or postpartum recovery.

A study from 2018 found that, at the time, women accounted for 42% of practicing psychiatrists, yet they held only 9% of senior academic leadership positions.[32] When the people with power haven't experienced something, it's far too easy for them to dismiss its importance.

The situation is equally dire when we look at training for OBGYNs. A 2024 article surveyed over 100 OBGYNs and found that over half had either no training in perinatal mental health or, at most, had attended one workshop on the subject.[33] These are physicians who will see thousands of pregnant and postpartum patients throughout their careers, and most of them had received virtually no formal education on the mental health complications they'd undoubtedly encounter along the way.

Dr. Jessica Vernon is an OBGYN who's now on the Board of PSI. She's also the author of the 2025 book *Then Comes Baby: An Honest Conversation about Birth, Postpartum, and the Complex Transition to Parenthood.* In a 2025 blog post for PSI, she shared that "my 'aha moment' came after my own struggle with postpartum anxiety, OCD, and depression… I had very little training during residency and was shocked when I started learning more about how pervasive and diverse PMADs [perinatal mood and anxiety disorders] are and can present in pregnant people and new parents."[34]

This echoes a trend I've noticed since I began speaking out about my experience with postpartum mental health struggles.

Those who seem to *really* care almost always have a personal experience driving their interest in the subject.[xxiv] While most people are kind and sympathetic toward me when I share my story, if I get serious interest or a follow-on conversation, it's almost assuredly followed by a reference to that person's personal experience, which is what enlightened them to the underground world of maternal mental health disorders and treatment.

I understand that, in some ways, this is just human nature: we're most interested in stories and issues we can personally relate to. But I also think we should expect better of ourselves as a society. We should care about fixing systemic problems even when they haven't touched us directly, especially when those systemic problems have dire consequences that aren't inevitable.

Thought exercise: Imagine if the number one complication of pregnancy was a painful, debilitating, and sometimes fatal (but highly treatable) parasitic infection that would afflict one

---

xxiv Including me! I didn't really pay any attention to maternal mental health until I experienced it. I'm not immune to this phenomenon.

in five new moms and set the child up for higher risk of a similar parasitic infection later in life.

I'm going to hazard a guess that most people, regardless of whether they'd seen this illness up close, would care about this complication and demand that we bolster our healthcare infrastructure to address it, including training all providers on the basics of how to recognize and respond to the infection. I imagine it wouldn't matter that OBGYNs aren't infectious disease doctors; they'd still brush up on the topic for the (extremely) likely scenario that they'd encounter a patient with said parasite.

I imagine we wouldn't leave it up to each individual doctor to decide whether or not they wanted to pursue more training on the issue. We would just universally require it, offer it, and find a way to make it happen.

After all, *of course* we would want to ensure we're doing everything we can to address the number one complication of childbirth, right?

I rest my case.

The knowledge gap among healthcare providers has significant consequences.

In the absence of perinatal mental health expertise, women sometimes elect, or are advised, to discontinue their psychiatric medications during pregnancy.

A study published in *JAMA Psychiatry* in 2025 found a large decrease in antidepressant use *without* an accompanying increase in psychotherapy during pregnancy, with antidepressant use returning to baseline about one month after delivery.[35] They inferred from this that a large population of women with active mental health conditions are going untreated during their pregnancy, which has consequences for both the mother and the baby. (More on this in Chapter 24.)

This knowledge gap also means that many women are given depression screenings at prenatal or postpartum appointments, only to be met with something akin to a blank stare when they disclose their mental health symptoms.

Speaking from personal experience, as I've stated before, this isn't just a missed opportunity. Those instances often add fuel to the fire; they are sending women the message that these conditions aren't important enough for their providers to know how to respond, or worse, that nothing can be done about them.

Making Some Progress

Fortunately, since the turn of the 21st century, a number of critical advances have helped to lay the groundwork for stronger education and training around maternal mental health.

In 2002, the first reproductive psychiatry training program was launched at the University of Illinois at Chicago, recognizing the need for specialized psychiatric care tailored to the unique mental health needs of people during their reproductive years. Fast-forward to 2026, and there are now 16 reproductive psychiatry subspecialty programs across the country.[36]

While this reflects remarkable progress and an encouraging trend, there's still a slight hitch: none of these fellowships are accredited by the Accreditation Council for Graduate Medical Education or formally recognized by the American Psychiatric Association. Without that institutional stamp of approval, many hospitals treat these fellowships as optional rather than essential, which is a critical barrier to broader adoption.[37]

In 2013, another major milestone occurred with the development of "The National Curriculum in Reproductive Psychiatry" (NCRP), a standardized educational resource designed to train residents and fellows in psychiatric and non-psychiatric specialties in this field.[38] A few years later, the group that created the NCRP partnered with Marcé of North America to merge and expand curriculum efforts, making it easier for clinicians and healthcare programs to access high-quality perinatal mental health education.[39]

In 2018, PSI launched the first certification program in perinatal mental health (PMH-C) for mental health professionals, including therapists, prescribers, and "affiliated professions" such as peer supporters, nurses, and doulas.[40] This has created a pathway for clinicians across disciplines to demonstrate specialized competence in perinatal mental health, helping to expand access to knowledgeable providers. PSI maintains a list of all certified providers on its website, and as of December 2025, there were over 7,000 non-expired PMH-C holders across 33 countries and territories around the world.[41]

In 2019, UMass Chan Medical School developed the Lifeline for Moms Perinatal Mental Health Toolkit to provide "actionable information, algorithms, and clinical pearls to support detection, assessment, and treatment of perinatal mood and anxiety disorders" for obstetric physicians.[42] This was released in collaboration with the American College of Obstetricians and Gynecologists and was supported by funding from the CDC.

Together, these developments signal an important cultural and clinical shift. They show that a growing number of people in medicine recognize that perinatal mental health is an important issue, and that it deserves the same attention and rigor we give to any other major health condition.

But we're still just at the beginning. Until every medical school and residency program *requires* perinatal mental health education, until every OBGYN and family medicine doctor graduates with competence in this field, and until we embed this knowledge into the standard curriculum rather than treating it as an elective add-on, we still have work to do.

At the end of the day, every pregnant person deserves to have access to evidence-based mental healthcare before, during, and after pregnancy. Not because they're lucky enough to find a provider who cares, and not because they stumbled upon the right specialist either in person or on social media, but because it's a standard, expected part of medical care.

CHAPTER 22

We're Missing the Infrastructure

When my family and I first met with Dr. E at the perinatal PHP, she explained the structure of the program to us and mentioned that it was one of only a few in the country.

As I began to recover and reflect on my experience, this started to seem odd. Along the way, I'd learned that experiences like mine (both the initial suffering part and the recovery-through-receiving-appropriate-care part) were common.

As a healthcare administrator, I found this particularly fascinating, so I dug in to unpack the entire care continuum for maternal mental health conditions, from lowest acuity to highest. Here's what I learned this care continuum looks like:

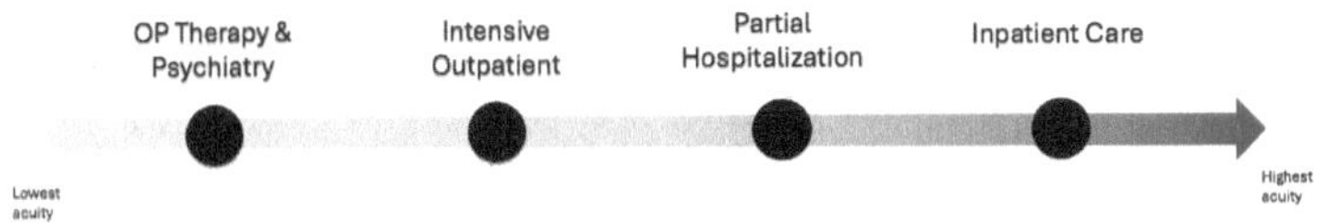

Outpatient Therapy and Psychiatry

On one end of the spectrum, there are outpatient therapists and psychiatrists with specialized training in perinatal care.

Unfortunately, even this lowest level of acuity, which theoretically should be the most accessible, is out of reach for most. A report published by the Policy Center for Maternal Mental Health in 2025 found that 84% of women live in maternal mental health "dark zones," meaning they live in an area with high need and low resource density.[43]

Intensive Outpatient Care

One step up on this ladder are intensive outpatient treatment programs, or IOPs. IOPs exist for many types of mental health needs, not just the perinatal population, and they offer more support than traditional one-to-one outpatient appointments.

Specialized *perinatal* IOPs are similar in structure yet vastly different in content from general adult IOPs for other mental health disorders. This is partly because perinatal IOPs are typically designed around the needs of mother–infant pairs, not just the mother alone. These programs, when they're offered in person, are equipped with baby gear and other amenities that allow a woman suffering from a mental health disorder to seek treatment while also caring for their infant. The providers who work in these programs have specific training in the perinatal period, and there's often "dyadic work" as part of the curriculum, which is focused on the relationship between the parent and the child.

It's also because the content and conversations in perinatal IOPs reflect the specific stage of life that pregnant and postpartum women are in. Conversations revolve around sleep deprivation, feeding struggles, poop explosions, and the seismic life transition associated with assuming responsibility for another human life, not just run-of-the-mill life stressors.

And just as important as the content of the conversations is the community. The group support component of IOPs is powerful, but it only works when participants feel understood and safe to share. For postpartum women, that means being surrounded by others who are also waking up every few hours, leaking through their shirts, and/or Googling "Is my baby supposed to breathe like that?" Talking with a middle-aged man who's struggling with unemployment or a young adult processing a breakup isn't the same. The community healing power of perinatal IOPs comes from sitting with other women who are walking through similar struggles, and who are also wondering whether becoming a mother has permanently broken something in them.

There are currently 39 perinatal IOPs nationwide, of which 12 are fully virtual. Of note, over half of those programs were established in the last five years (since 2021).

The 27 in-person programs are spread across 16 states plus D.C. I'm a bit of an Excel nerd, so I created an algorithm to calculate how far individuals in each zip code are from their nearest in-person perinatal IOP. I used population data from the CDC and the latitude/longitude coordinates of each existing in-person program.

In my estimation, few people can (or should be expected to) drive more than 25 miles to attend an in-person program that meets several times a week, especially for a condition this common. It's an arbitrary cutoff, but I think it's a fair one, particularly for this population.

Moms with severe depression might find it challenging just to get out of bed and get dressed in the morning. A short drive might be doable, but each additional mile adds to the activation energy—already in short supply—required to attend treatment. For those with postpartum anxiety or OCD, the barriers can look different but feel just as paralyzing. Many feel compelled to stop and check on their baby every few minutes. Some don't feel comfortable driving at all.

I was in the latter camp. When I was sick, I could drive myself short distances, but I was terrified of driving with my baby. I didn't trust myself to drive him to the grocery store, let alone into the city where the program was located. My mom or my husband drove me to treatment every day.

And I'm not the only one.

A young single mom I met in my program who was battling bipolar disorder and severe anxiety took a 20-plus-mile taxi ride with her baby each day to attend treatment. I once spoke with a woman whose husband drove her, doing a round trip both ways, to a perinatal PHP more than an hour away from their home. In other words, he spent over four hours in the car each day, for weeks on end, so that she could attend.

If accessing care requires that level of coordination and privilege, then for much of the population, it might as well not exist.

Using my distance calculations, I found that only 16% of women aged 15–50 live within 25 miles of an existing perinatal IOP, while 84% do not.

This does not mean that 16% of women actually have access to this kind of care, because there are more factors at play when it comes to healthcare access than distance alone: insurance coverage, time off, childcare, transportation, program capacity, etc.

But my calculations demonstrate that 16% is the *maximum* percentage of American women of reproductive age with access to this form of care, because only 16% of that population even lives anywhere near a specialized program.

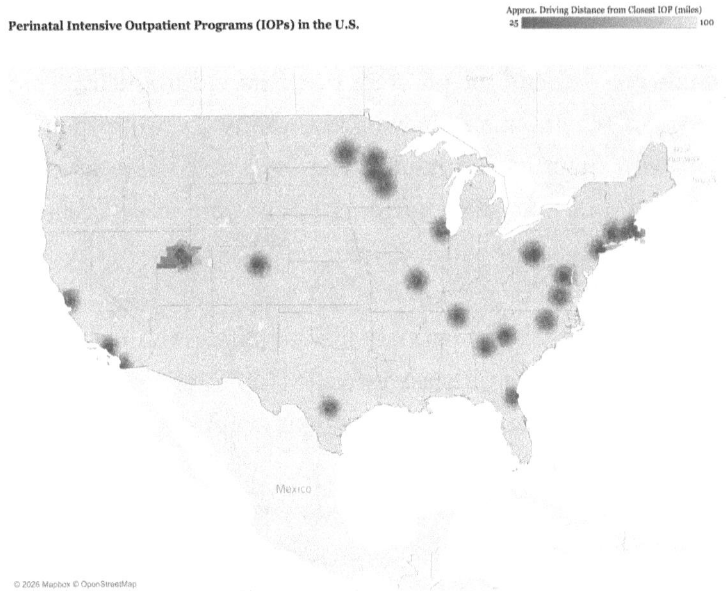

Figure 1: A map of in-person perinatal intensive outpatient programs throughout the United States, created by Emily Johnson using Tableau. Information about the data used to create these maps can be found at the end of the chapter. More information on these programs can be found in the Appendix.

Partial Hospitalization Programs (PHPs)

The next step up in intensity is a PHP. Similar to perinatal IOPs, perinatal PHPs are similar in concept to adult PHPs but are tailored toward the unique needs of pregnant and postpartum moms, not the least of which is the ability to whip out a boob in the middle of a session if needed if they're breastfeeding but haven't yet unlocked the expert-level status required to do this discreetly beneath a nursing cover.

The first-ever perinatal PHP in the U.S. opened at Women & Infants Hospital in Rhode Island in 2000.[44] A study of this program published over 10 years ago, in 2014, looked at 800 patient satisfaction surveys; it found that 97% of respondents agreed that the program had been helpful to them and 99% would recommend the program to others. Additionally, women often remarked that having the ability to bring their infant with them to treatment was a "welcomed feature of the program and that being surrounded by women experiencing similar concerns provides much-needed support and reduces isolation."[45]

Okay, okay, so patients *like* the program… but we can't invest in expensive healthcare infrastructure just because moms *like* the experience, some cynics might say. Are these programs clinically effective?

The answer to this is a resounding yes.

Another study published in 2021 looked at screening scores for over 300 women admitted to the Mother-Baby Day Hospital at Hennepin Healthcare in Minnesota, another perinatal PHP that was founded in 2013. The researchers found statistically significant improvements in scores on three different clinical outcome measures: the EPDS, the Generalized Anxiety Disorder 7-item scale, and the Barking Index of Maternal Functioning.[46]

Depression scores dropped from an average of 19 to 12, anxiety scores dropped from 15 to 9, and maternal functioning scores increased from 69 to 87. In other words, on average, this program reduced new mothers' depression scores from moderate/severe down to mild,[47] and anxiety scores from moderate/severe down to mild/moderate.[48]

I'm not a mental health professional, so don't take this too literally, but as someone who's been through this, I'd describe these changes in terms of my own journey as follows:

- **Depression:** Going from "living in black and white, physically and mentally unable to read their baby book" to "occasionally has bad days, but is generally able to participate in normal life, feel joy at milestones, and look forward to what lies ahead."
- **Anxiety:** Going from "limited appetite, upset gastrointestinal system, checking the baby for breathing eight times while driving five minutes to the grocery store" to "still occasionally nervous while the baby sleeps, but able to drive five minutes without checking for proof of life."

Programs like these exist in other parts of the world as well, with similar results. A study of a Mother-Baby Day Hospital (MBDH) at Clinic Barcelona in Spain found that "at discharge, *100% of women no longer met the full criteria for the main diagnosis.*" They found significant improvements in depression and anxiety symptoms, mother–infant bonding, and functional impairment, which were also seen at three-month follow-up. The MBDH was rated by mothers as an excellent-quality program, and they would recommend it.[49]

A quarter of a century after the first perinatal PHP opened in Rhode Island, we're sitting at a grand total of eight such programs in the United States. Here's what that looks like:

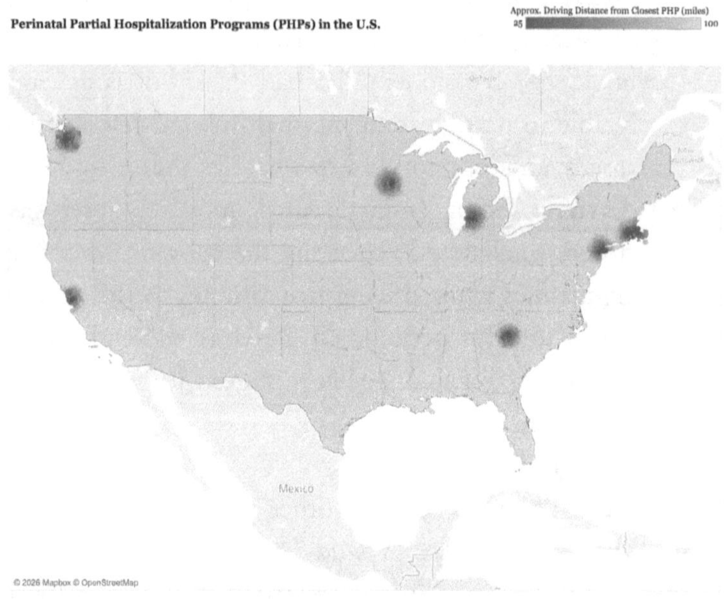

Figure 2: A map of perinatal PHPs throughout the United States, created by Emily Johnson using Tableau. Information about the data used to create these maps can be found at the end of the chapter. More information on these programs can be found in the Appendix.

I did a similar exercise with Excel and population data to the one I did with IOPs, and I found that only 7% of women aged 15–50 live within 25 miles of a perinatal PHP; 93% do not.

Again, this means that 7% is the *upper limit* on who has access to programs like this: the actual number is much less than that once you account for barriers related to coverage, time off, childcare, and so on.

Inpatient Care

The final step up the ladder is inpatient care. In several other countries around the world, such as the UK, France, Australia, New Zealand, India, and Sri Lanka, this often means inpatient care on a mother–baby joint admission unit (MBU), where the mother and the baby are admitted together. Strengthening the relationship between the two is recognized as an important part of the treatment; conversely, separating them is recognized as clinically harmful.[50]

But here in the United States, we have a habit of being stingy when it comes to types of healthcare not frequently (or ever) needed by commercially insured men. So, someone once decreed that admitting a physically healthy infant alongside their mother would be an unnecessary expense;[51] thus, this model of care doesn't exist here.

There's only one other argument I've heard about why we don't have, and don't even seem to entertain the concept of, mother–baby psychiatric units in the U.S., and that's the issue of liability. Why admit a healthy baby if doing so introduces the possibility of that baby getting hurt or contracting a hospital-acquired infection, which poses a liability to the hospital?

My thoughts on this are similar to my thoughts on the sleep and feeding questions, which is that context matters, and it matters quite a bit.

Yes, admitting a physically healthy baby to any kind of medical facility introduces the risk of that baby getting hurt somehow or contracting a hospital-acquired infection. Of course, there are things we could do to minimize those risks as much as possible, but some level of risk will always remain.

But those risks must be weighed against the alternative, which for some babies is one or more of the following, all of which are known to be adverse childhood events:[52]

- Being removed (potentially permanently) from their mother.
- Being cared for at home by a severely ill mother who knows hospitalization simply isn't an option for her,

> because she doesn't have any trusted and/or available people nearby to care for her baby.
> - Being cared for at home by the non-birthing parent, who then loses their job once they exhaust their allowed time off, leading to financial insecurity and exposure to poverty.

Worst of all, the risk of infanticide among mothers with untreated postpartum psychosis is 4%.[53]

When you begin to weigh these actual scenarios, the answer to which one is better for the baby (hospital admission or no hospital admission) is far less straightforward.

I was lucky: I had a husband with time off and family nearby to step in. However, that is not the reality for all women. We need to build systems that work for *most* people, not just a lucky few.

While we do not have what many people internationally consider to be the gold standard of treatment for severely ill perinatal women (MBUs), some tireless advocates in the U.S. have found a way to come pretty darn close.

In 2011, the first-ever perinatal psychiatry unit (parent-admission only) opened at the University of North Carolina Chapel Hill.[54] Today, to my knowledge, there are five such units, randomly scattered throughout the country.

Here is an exhaustive list of where you should try to be located if you happen to need round-the-clock psychiatric care during your pregnancy or postpartum journey (which, by the way, can happen to literally anybody who becomes pregnant, with little to no warning):[55]

- Chapel Hill, NC
- Little Rock, AR
- Baton Rouge, LA
- Mountain View, CA
- New York City, NY[56]

Or, visually:

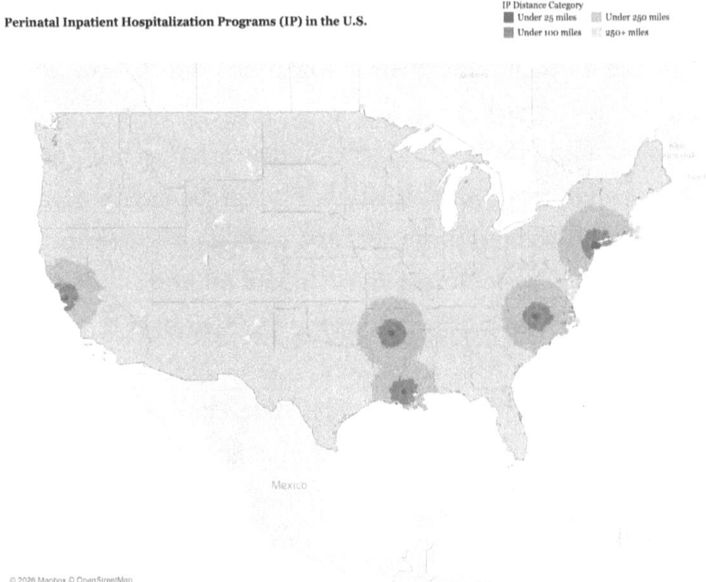

Figure 3: A map of perinatal inpatient units throughout the United States, created by Emily Johnson using Tableau. Information about the data used to create these maps can be found at the end of the chapter. More information on these programs can be found in the Appendix.

Even if you are in one of these places, just to be on the safe side, I suggest you take a screenshot of the program list in the Appendix. It's highly unlikely that the doctors you interact with in the OB clinic or the ER will know to direct you toward the perinatal psychiatry unit in your area rather than a general one.

I adjusted the color coding a little bit for this map, recognizing that some people probably have a higher tolerance for driving longer distances to reach inpatient services, since it doesn't require a daily commute for the person receiving care. That being said, traveling over 100 miles by car is likely prohibitive for many (if not most).

The Royal College of Psychiatrists in the UK recommends having one eight-bedded MBU per 15,000 deliveries.[57] In the UK, they have 22 MBUs,[58] about half of what that benchmark would recommend for their population, which sees about 700,000 deliveries/year.

In the U.S., we have 3.6 million deliveries/year. Using the international standard, that would suggest we have a need for 240 MBUs throughout the country. Even if we're comfortable substituting adult-only perinatal inpatient units for MBUs, we only have five out of the recommended 240. Or, in other words, about 2% of what we need.

It's certainly possible that we could develop a better continuum of care that necessitates fewer inpatient units in the U.S. than they use in the UK: more preventive care, more outpatient programs, and so on. But even if that would allow us to cut the number of inpatient units needed by half, we would *still* be short more than 100 specialized psychiatric inpatient units.

So... What's the Deal?

Back to the question I posed in the introduction to this book: given the prevalence of maternal mental health disorders and the impact they have on maternal morbidity and mortality, and given the research suggesting that specialized intensive treatment programs like the one I attended have a remarkable impact on symptoms, *how on Earth do we only have a handful throughout the country?*

As with many things, it really comes down to how we finance healthcare in the United States.

An article about the perinatal PHP in Rhode Island notes that "this treatment model has proven to be successful and financially sustainable for over a decade." That might sound great on the surface, but programs like that often require significant up-front capital investments for both the physical setup and program design. For example, the most recent perinatal inpatient unit that opened in Louisiana reportedly cost eight million dollars to build.[59]

Unfortunately, my experience suggests that nobody in healthcare leadership is racing to build new programs that are at best going to be described as "sustainable." To get a CEO interested in using capital dollars for an investment that isn't legally required of you, you typically need to be showing projections of double-digit ROIs.

Most of those C-suite leaders, regardless of the ideology they purport, will choose a new dermatology clinic or a new same-day-surgery center *any day* over a women's mental health program.

I would be remiss if I didn't also offer their perspective, which is that (nonprofit) hospital margins in this day and age are actually quite slim[60] and are threatening to get worse by the year. Nonprofit health system CEOs are not chasing flashy, high-yield investments because it pads their personal pockets (most of the time). They're choosing them because they think those investments offer their health system a better chance at long-term viability.

I get that perspective; I really do.

And I'm also not afraid to admit that, regardless of rationale, the outcome is the same.

Keep an eye on your local newspapers to see what kinds of new healthcare facilities (if any) are going up around you. I'm willing to bet that, more often than not, it's a high-tech imaging, same-day surgery, dermatology center or the like (with some primary care offices thrown in, because you can't forget to build the pipeline for the aforementioned high-yield services).

To underscore what it actually takes to build and sustain one of the few intensive perinatal programs that exists today, I asked Paige Bellenbaum, a licensed therapist, healthcare leader, and founding member of New York's only perinatal PHP, to share her perspective. Like most of the change-makers I've encountered in this space, she came to work in this area as a result of lived experience.

Expert Perspective: The Staggering Gaps in Perinatal Mental Healthcare

By: Paige Bellenbaum, LCSW, PMH-C
Perinatal Mental Health Specialist, Paige Bellenbaum Consulting
Adjunct Professor, Silberman School of Social Work, Hunter College
Advanced Perinatal Psychotherapy Trainer, Postpartum Support International
Education and Government Relations Consultant, The Motherhood Center

For nearly two decades, I've worked in the field of perinatal mental health, and I can honestly say we've seen tremendous progress. Public awareness has grown, screening has become more routine, and providers increasingly recognize perinatal mood and anxiety disorders (PMADs).

Yet the gap between clinical need and available services remains staggering, especially for those with severe symptoms.

Let's explore mental health through a physical health lens. If someone hurts their ankle, there are a range of injuries. A sprain might require ice packs or an ACE bandage, a fracture might require a brace or crutches, and a break might require surgery and extensive physical therapy. For women experiencing PMADs, mild symptoms might respond well to therapy and/or support groups, while moderate symptoms might respond well to medication or a perinatal intensive outpatient program. For severe symptoms, a perinatal partial hospital program or inpatient hospitalization may be required. Symptoms of severe depression, suicidality, or psychosis cannot be safely managed in standard outpatient care, just as a broken ankle can't be managed with an ice pack.

I was an original founding member of The Motherhood Center in 2017. Our goal at the time was simple but ambitious: to fill a glaring gap in the continuum of care for the perinatal population. We created New York's first and only licensed perinatal PHP: a Day Program where new and expecting mothers could receive intensive treatment for moderate to severe PMADs while keeping their babies close. Since its inception, The Motherhood Center has treated thousands of women in the Day Program, helping them return to baseline functioning and feel connected to their babies.

On average, participants entered the Day Program with an EPDS score above 18 (consistent with major depression) and were discharged with a score below 9. In other words, most women cut their depression scores by more than half over the course of treatment.

Many said the same words at discharge: "This program saved my life."

So, why aren't there more programs like this one?

First, they're **resource-intensive**. Perinatal programs require doctors and clinicians trained in reproductive psychiatry, specialized perinatal therapy, and dyadic care. On-site nursery space and services, baby supplies, and staff who can safely support both mother and infant all add cost. Yet there is no dedicated billing code for perinatal IOPs or PHPs, meaning programs must rely on generic reimbursement rates for higher levels of care that don't reflect this added complexity.

Second, **funding is scarce**. Public investment has largely focused on awareness and screening, which are vital but insufficient when there's nowhere to send a perinatal person who's experiencing a PMAD. There have been little to no federal initiatives aimed at expanding higher-level treatment nationwide, and even the programs that are fortunate enough to launch often struggle to survive given inadequate reimbursement rates.

Third, **the workforce gap** is real. There simply aren't enough clinicians trained in reproductive psychiatry and perinatal treatment to staff programs at scale. Building that pipeline requires targeted investment in training and education as well.

Despite these challenges, the outcomes speak for themselves. Intensive programs help mothers recover and strengthen attachment with their babies. They reduce the risk of suicide (the leading cause of maternal death in the U.S.) and support family stability. And untreated PMAD illness has a $14.2 billion price tag annually, so there's a financial incentive as well.

We know what works. What's missing is the infrastructure to make it accessible and the funding to make that possible.

Expanding access to intensive perinatal programs will require:

- Dedicated CPT codes[xxv] and fair reimbursement rates for perinatal-specific care
- Federal and state funding to develop perinatal IOP and PHP programs in high-need regions
- Investment in workforce training to expand the pipeline of clinicians with perinatal expertise
- Integration of intensive perinatal treatment into maternal health policy as an essential component of care

Perinatal mental healthcare should not depend on where someone lives or how much they can pay. It should be part of a robust nationwide system that meets mothers wherever they are on the spectrum of need. We have the evidence, the models, and the will. What remains is the collective decision to build the infrastructure that mothers and their babies need and deserve.

Data Notes

To create the distance calculations, I used program addresses from individual program websites and population data from the U.S. Census Bureau.[61] Driving distances are approximate based on latitude/longitude data, applying a reasonable conversion factor to estimate driving distance from the straight-line distance between coordinates.[62]

---

xxv Current procedural terminology (CPT) codes are numbers used in the U.S. healthcare system to identify medical services and procedures delivered by qualified healthcare professionals.

CHAPTER 23

This Is Not a New Problem

Is the lack of training and resources on this topic because the existence or frequency of maternal mental health disorders is a new phenomenon?

No. Not even a little bit.

Again, I'll share some anecdotal evidence as well as some published evidence. The purpose of this chapter is not to give an in-depth explanation of the history of postpartum mental illness and its treatment. For anyone interested in that, I'd recommend checking out *Motherhood and Mental Illness* by Emma Hayes or *Blue: A History of Postpartum Depression in America* by Rachel Moran.

Instead, the purpose of this chapter is to give you just a taste of that history: enough to show you that maternal mental health disorders are not some new phenomenon created by "lazy and entitled millennial moms" or "even lazier and more entitled Gen Z moms."

The Anecdotal Stuff

When I started publicly sharing my story, people, mostly women, started to come out of the woodwork with their own stories or stories about people they knew.

A relative of my husband shared that one of her high school classmates died by suicide in the 1960s, just a few months after giving birth, and that she speculated the same thing may have happened to another one of her classmates. She also shared a story of a close friend who was hospitalized shortly after her second child was born, receiving mental health treatments that resulted in severe memory loss.

Next, a relative of mine casually shared in conversation, "Oh, when Bobby was born, I had the strangest thoughts. I thought he was an alien sent by God to torture me."

In other words, she probably just white-knuckled it through postpartum psychosis, a medical emergency. Cool.

Another admitted that she had "bad thoughts," and each time they popped up, she'd "stop what she was doing and pray to God for them to go away."

Okay, so perhaps there's a genetic predisposition to this in my family. That would've been nice to know a little sooner.

At a conference I attended, which was unrelated to maternal mental health, a female leader of a large corporation confided in me (via whisper, not-so-subtly revealing her deep shame about the topic) that she, too, had suffered from postpartum depression, and that in fact her aunt had died by suicide after her cousin was born.

Another woman, at this same conference, shared with me that her mother had been hospitalized on general psychiatric units for *a total of 15 months* between multiple pregnancies: a fact that her mother disclosed to her only after she had a child of her own and started vocalizing some mental health challenges.

I was stunned.

But at the same time, I wasn't. By talking publicly and matter-of-factly about maternal mental health, I seem to have unlocked a door for people to openly share things that are otherwise hidden in their closet of family secrets.

At this point, it's something I've simply come to expect; it's that common. These conditions aren't new, although the frequency of them might be increasing. People just haven't had words for them and/or felt safe to talk about them.

Non-anecdotal Evidence

But you don't have to just take my word for it.

In her book *Motherhood and Mental Illness*, psychologist Emma Hayes shares that the history of female hysteria dates back to Ancient Egypt, around 1,900 B.C.E. This hysteria was thought to be attributable to "malaise of the uterus," and cures included smelling salts and, my favorite, "fulfillment of inadequate sex life and procreation."[63] In other words, they thought perhaps the cure for mental illness in women was to have *more* children.

Hayes also says that "throughout the ages there has been a known link between insanity and childbirth, with even Queen Victoria experiencing a period of low mood after the birth of her second child, documented in 1841, which then recurred after each of her subsequent seven pregnancies."[64] To me, this is a reminder both that postpartum depression has been around for a long time and that it can affect anyone, regardless of their social status or relative wealth.

In 1839, a physician named Robert Gooch published a book called *An Account of Some of the Most Important Diseases Peculiar to Women*. It includes a chapter called "Disorders of the mind in lying-in women," which details the cases of several postpartum women he worked with in his career with "mania" or "melancholia."[65]

In the more recent past, the term "postpartum depression" appeared in *Good Housekeeping* magazine in 1960. The article, titled "Those Mysterious Childbirth Blues," said, "When a woman goes into an apparently causeless state of depression ... chances are she is having an attack of 'third-day blues', 'childbirth blues', or what doctors call 'postpartum depression.'"[66]

The Rolling Stones song "Mother's Little Helper" came out in 1966, referencing tranquilizers that had recently come out and were becoming popular among housewives. The song, as I interpret it, implies that the women taking it were not actually sick.

Let's pause there for a moment and reflect on the term "causeless" from the magazine article and the insinuation that mothers taking anxiety medications in the 1960s weren't really sick.

"Causeless" in reference to postpartum depression is an interesting descriptor, given that childbirth is a major medical and life event that also often happens to coincide with the largest sudden drop in hormones a human can or will ever experience. And perhaps some women taking Valium in the 1960s weren't really ill, but I'd bet many of them truly were, at a time when there were very few tools available to help them manage their symptoms (again, despite this being a recognized issue for millennia).

Why do several of these references both acknowledge mental health issues among mothers and invalidate them in the same breath? Perhaps because until at least the 1980s, the leading "voices" on this topic were men. For more on that and the history of advocacy in this space, I'd recommend checking out Moran's book.

In summary, maternal mental health disorders are not new. And they're certainly not a reflection of modern-day women's inability to handle the rigors of parenthood. Pregnancy, childbirth, and postpartum are vulnerable times for mental health. The fact that this is true, and that we still do such a poor job of treating these conditions, is a reflection on how much stock we put in women's pain and suffering.

We can't change the past. We can't go back in time and offer compassionate, effective treatment to the millions of moms who've suffered or died prematurely as a result of the callous nature with which these disorders have been handled by the medical field.

But we sure as hell can change the future.

CHAPTER 24

Why Does This Matter Again?

I hope that it's abundantly clear by now why all of these things (the gaps in training, the gaps in infrastructure, the swaths of women who are suffering without treatment) matter. But if not, I want to conclude by offering some data on the implications of what I've laid out in this book.

Let's do a few quick math exercises using well-cited statistics on the prevalence of maternal mental health disorders (and if you're not interested in the math and are willing to take my word for it, just glance through the bolded lines).

<u>Quantity of Suffering</u>
3.6 million live births per year in the U.S. ×
20% prevalence of maternal mental health disorders

= 720,000 women suffering from maternal mental health disorders each year

I'll use this number as our baseline, although it's an understatement, because you can develop maternal mental health disorders whether or not your pregnancy led to a live birth. Then:

> 720,000 women with maternal mental health disorders ×
> 75% untreated

> **= 540,000 women with maternal mental health disorders go untreated each year**

In other words, over half a million American women suffer from untreated maternal mental health disorders each year.

Quantity of Loss

To estimate how many lives are lost each year to maternal mental health disorders, let's start with our maternal mortality rate, though this statistic only measures deaths that occur during delivery through 42 days postpartum.

> 3.6 million births per year in the U.S. ×
> 19 in 100,000 maternal mortality rate[67]

> **= 684 maternal deaths from birth through 42 days postpartum**

But we know that 30% of all maternal deaths occur from 43 days to one year postpartum, so we'll have to adjust this number to account for that.

> 684 deaths /
> 1-0.3 (the percentage of maternal deaths that occur
> from 43 days to one year postpartum)

= 977 maternal deaths/year when looking at birth to one year postpartum

Now that we have an estimate of the true number of maternal deaths each year, we can apply what we know about the percentage of those deaths that are attributable to mental health disorders.

977 deaths/year ×
22.7% of deaths attributed to maternal mental health disorders[68]

= 222 women/year lost to maternal suicide or overdose from birth to one year postpartum

Almost all, if not all, of those represent preventable deaths.

The Impact Is Multigenerational

If you aren't moved by the pain and suffering experienced by women, perhaps you'll be moved by the pain and suffering this causes their babies.

Research consistently shows that untreated maternal mental health disorders have profound physical and mental health impacts on the babies caught in the mix. Women with untreated mental health conditions have a higher risk of preterm birth and of having babies with low birth weight.[69] Babies born to women with untreated maternal mental health conditions are also predisposed to having mental health struggles of their own, both in infancy and throughout their lives.[70] The Zero To Three Foundation, a nonprofit focused on early childhood development, describes how parents' mental health can impact their young children through in utero cortisol exposure, epigenetic changes, and ability to provide attuned parenting.[71]

Julian was fortunate enough, I hope, to avoid feeling the full effects of my illness due to (relatively) quick intervention and limitless family support. But research would suggest that he didn't come through unscathed.

As psychologist Catherine Monk from Columbia University explains, research on children ages four to thirteen found that high maternal anxiety during pregnancy "predicted a doubling of children's risk for behavioral health problems such as ADHD and anxiety." Similar evidence exists for untreated maternal stress and depression.[72]

Looking back on my pregnancy, it's clear I had untreated anxiety throughout.

When my confidence in speaking so publicly on this topic wanes (and, believe me, it often does), one of the things that inevitably brings me back to a level of productive rage is knowing that because of my untreated anxiety in pregnancy, Julian carries a higher risk of anxiety in his life. And as I know now, anxiety is not just a nuisance or a silly personality quirk; it can be debilitating, if not outright dangerous. This risk was bestowed upon him before he took his first breath, because the U.S. healthcare system was not adequately prepared to protect his mother and, by extension, him.

A Vicious Cycle

Zooming out to a macro level, I don't think it's particularly political to state that it really feels like our country is falling apart at the seams in terms of mental health. In 2022, suicide was the 11th leading cause of death,[73] responsible for nearly 50,000 deaths.

For most of us, it's even *more* gut-wrenching to think about the state of children's mental health. Anxiety and depression rates have risen among young people over the last decade, worsened by the 2020–2023 pandemic. In 2023, the CDC found that two in ten (20%) high school students had seriously considered attempting suicide, and nearly one in ten (9%) had actually attempted it.[74]

WHAT?

Read those numbers again.

If they seem implausible, as they would've seemed to me before I had an experiential crash course in mental health, you might be surprised to learn that suicide is the second leading cause of death among children between the ages of 10 and 14 and the third leading cause among people aged 15–24.[75]

"Okay, that's horrible," you might be thinking, "but what does it have to do with maternal mental health?"

Well, studies suggest that one of the most significant risk factors for developing maternal mental health disorders like postpartum depression is a history of depression.[76]

Let's connect some dots:

Untreated maternal mental health disorders increase the risk of mental health disorders in kids,

 ↳ which increases the prevalence of maternal mental health disorders for the next generation of parents,

  ↳ which increases the risk of mental health disorders in the subsequent generation of kids,

   ↳ and so on.

We're stuck in a vicious cycle.

Investing heavily in new mothers is one way to break it.

The Economic Case

Before moving forward, I want to drive home the importance of addressing maternal mental health disorders for even the most skeptical or misogynistic among us, who might not be moved by the plight of women or children alone. So, here is some economic rationale for why everyone should care about the lack of maternal mental health infrastructure.

In 2020, the *American Journal of Public Health* published a study estimating the average cost of untreated maternal mental health conditions, accounting for higher maternal healthcare expenditures, reduced economic productivity, and increased childhood healthcare expenditures attributable to these disorders.

The cost? Approximately $32,000 per mother–infant dyad, totaling **$14 billion annually.**[77]

Candidly, I'm not sure how much it would cost in terms of infrastructure investments to move the needle on this issue. But I'm confident it's far less than the $140 billion we should expect untreated maternal mental health disorders to cost our country over the next decade.

Morals aside, investing in this kind of infrastructure is an economic no-brainer.

But insurance companies play a big role in the success—or lack thereof—of healthcare transformation in this area. Unless they compensate adequately for this kind of care, these programs will cease to exist, regardless of their efficacy. And insurance companies don't care about macro-level societal costs, the cynic might say. Does this really impact *their* bottom line?

Yes.

A 2022 study analyzing hospital delivery claims found that childbirth hospitalizations for mothers with mental health disorders had 50% higher rates of severe maternal morbidity and $458 higher average costs: an estimated $102 million in additional annual U.S. costs, primarily borne by employers and Medicaid.[78]

In other words, payers will be shelling out over one billion dollars in *excess delivery costs alone* over the next decade as a result of untreated mental health disorders among pregnant women. That doesn't even include the downstream costs to insurance companies, of which there are many (psychiatric hospitalizations, increased pediatric ER utilization, etc.).[79]

Anecdotally, I can also confirm that my insurance company paid a heck of a lot more in the long run for my mental health-care by allowing it to reach a crisis point before I got connected to anyone with a modicum of expertise on the topic.

I was lucky. I was in an inpatient general hospital unit for "only" three nights, because of my mom's miraculous discovery of a perinatal PHP that allowed me and my family to feel good about my discharge plan.

That three-day inpatient hospital stay, which introduced a whole new level of trauma to my journey, cost my health insurance company nearly $9,000 (and that's what they actually paid, not just what the hospital charged).[xxvi]

I know women who've been hospitalized for weeks or months. One of those women is someone I'll call Katie, a friend of mine from the perinatal PHP I attended. She was also battling perinatal OCD, but unfortunately it took longer for that to be identified and appropriately treated for her. She recently allowed me to look through her claims data with her, and here's what we found.

---

xxvi A funny-money concept that nobody, even those with advanced degrees in the field, seem to be able to truly justify.

Katie's Story, and the Actual Financial Cost of Systemic Failure

As a refresher, perinatal OCD is a sneaky son-of-a-bitch. Characterized by intrusive thoughts that cause significant distress paired with compulsive actions to alleviate that distress, it often hides behind a façade of normalcy. Who wants to volunteer that they've had terrifying thoughts about driving off a bridge or about harming their healthy baby? Nobody.

Perinatal OCD preys on your deepest fears and inserts doubt where it doesn't belong.

In hindsight, my friend Katie had several telltale signs of postpartum OCD from the beginning.

When her baby was about a month old, Katie began to have intrusive thoughts about harming herself, which were confusing and deeply distressing to her. These thoughts scared her so much that she asked her husband to hide the knives in the kitchen and anything else she could use to hurt herself.

Over time, the distress intensified. What started as uncomfortable but manageable spiraled into paralyzing fear as Katie wondered if this was her permanent reality. A few months in, believing she was a danger to herself, she voluntarily went to a local ER.

The ER provider asked Katie if she was thinking about harming herself or her baby, to which Katie, a self-described "rule follower" who was actively in search of help for these intrusive thoughts, answered honestly: "Yes, constantly."

Interpreting this (incorrectly) as a sign of suicidal ideation and severe depression rather than as the symptom of OCD that it was, Katie was separated from her family and admitted to the hospital's general inpatient psychiatric unit, where she stayed for the next 12 days.

The unit had no private rooms, so staff advised against having her family bring her newborn baby to visit. A kind nurse on the unit, recognizing the harm that this would likely cause a new mom, advocated for an exception. During Katie's 12-day stay, her baby was allowed to visit twice, for one hour each time, in a separate room.

Katie spent her days calling her husband repeatedly ("What clothes did you put her in?" "Has she made any new noises?"), trying to stay connected to her family while sitting alone in a psychiatric unit.

Within days of her admission, a provider recommended electroconvulsive therapy (ECT), an invasive treatment involving electrical currents passed through the brain to induce seizure under general anesthesia.[xxvii] Desperate for relief and willing to do anything for her baby and family, Katie agreed. Just five days after arriving at the ER, and before ever being evaluated by a perinatal psychiatrist, she began a series of 12 ECT treatments.

ECT had little impact on her symptoms, so Katie continued to seek help. She tried everything from GeneSight testing to physical medicine to ketamine therapy, eventually landing in the perinatal PHP where we met.

By this point, Katie was experiencing some symptoms of anxiety and depression too, so they became the focus. Once again, the underlying OCD at the root of her illness was missed.

All told, Katie was hospitalized in a general psychiatric unit three separate times during her baby's first year, for a total of nearly a month.

---

xxvii ECT is an evidence-based treatment for some forms of depression, but not a first-line treatment for perinatal OCD.

What	Days	Amount Paid by Insurance
General inpatient stay 1 + ECT	12	$48,217
General inpatient stay 2	12	$18,527
General inpatient stay 3	5	$9,533
Total	29	$76,277

In total, her health insurance company paid over $76,000 for these hospitalizations and treatments. And again, this is what they *actually* paid; the amount "charged" by the hospital was nearly three times more.

Katie believes that much, if not all, of this could have been prevented had a single provider mentioned the term "perinatal OCD" when she first disclosed her symptoms.

While insurance bore the financial burden of these hospital bills, Katie and her family incurred significant financial costs, too. Her husband had to take additional, unplanned time off work. They scrambled to find last-minute childcare for their daughter so that he could return. Securing emergency childcare is no small feat in a country where daycare waiting lists sometimes exceed a year, so they settled on a daycare 15 minutes away that cost nearly $500/week.

But the financial costs, though real and significant, pale against the emotional toll of our current reality.

When we reviewed her treatment timeline and claims data, I watched sadness cross Katie's face as she recounted learning from her mother via phone, while sitting alone in a psychiatric unit, that her daughter had learned to crawl.

That's just one milestone of many that she'll never get back. Now, Katie carries not just the trauma of hospitalization but the grief of those lost moments, all because the system wasn't equipped to recognize or treat perinatal OCD, a relatively common and treatable condition.

Katie isn't an anomaly, any more than I am. Right now, at this very moment, there are probably hundreds, if not more, postpartum women in the U.S. locked in general psychiatric units, away from their babies, receiving inadequate care from undertrained providers.

The $76,000 that Katie's health plan paid for unnecessary hospitalizations and procedures represents not just wasted spending but lost milestones, accumulated trauma, and the compounding costs of a system that doesn't just fail to prevent suffering but actively adds to it.

A system that isn't designed to recognize or treat perinatal mental health conditions costs everyone, no matter how you measure it.

CHAPTER 25

Let's Dream Together for a Moment

That last chapter was a downer. I know that. I'm sorry.

But, as I've said before, and as I'll keep saying for the rest of my time on Earth, the miracle here that keeps me going is that maternal mental health conditions are treatable.

So, while our current reality is a sad one, there's reason to be hopeful about the future.

Let me paint a picture for you:

A world in which there are enough perinatal therapists and specialized treatment programs in every major city, so that a woman's chance (and that of her baby) at surviving and fully recovering from a psychiatric emergency doesn't depend on whether she lives in Providence, Rhode Island (where there's an intensive program) or Houston, Texas (where there isn't).

A world in which all women are screened for signs of mental health disorders during pregnancy and throughout their first year postpartum, and where OBGYNs, midwives, pediatricians, and family medicine doctors truly buy in to this process, because they know exactly what to do and where to point her in the event that she screens positive for an issue that requires treatment.

A world in which no woman is given advice to automatically discontinue her depression or anxiety medication simply because she's pregnant, not realizing that the risks to the baby of exposure to medication need to be weighed against the risks to the baby of exposure to untreated mental health disorders.

A world in which pregnant and postpartum women being treated for psychiatric illness (for perhaps the very first time) are treated by psychiatrists or other prescribers with formal training in perinatal psychiatry rather than by those with little to no formal training in this area, who often inadvertently make women feel worse than they did before seeking treatment.

A world in which the U.S. maternal mortality rate drops significantly because we've nearly eliminated maternal suicide and decreased pregnancy complications such as pre-eclampsia, C-section deliveries, and prolonged labors, which all open the door to additional complications.[80]

A world in which we don't stop there, at strong mental health support for birthing mothers of live babies. A world where we also have robust infrastructure in place to support new dads/non-birthing partners, people struggling with infertility, and people who've experienced loss, all of whom also have an elevated risk of mental health issues but would not be appropriately served by this ideal maternal mental health structure even if it were in place today.

A world in which, for the first time in a long time, the mental health of the next generation is stronger than the mental health of their parents and grandparents.

I believe all of this is possible.

We just have to decide, collectively, that this is the future that we want, and that this is the future we want badly enough that we're willing to invest in it using our time, attention, and money.

Feedback that's simply critical and doesn't offer ideas on how to improve has always been a huge pet peeve of mine, so I always strive to meet criticism with suggestions whenever humanly possible.

Here's a roadmap of what that might look like depending on what role you play in the lives of reproductive people. There's repetition in here, because this roadmap has been built to allow you to skip directly to the section that's most relevant to you.

"What Can YOU do?" Action Roadmap

If you're a survivor…

- Be kind to yourself. You didn't ask to be part of this club, and what you went through was not your fault. If you still feel like it was your fault despite me saying that it wasn't, see the next bullet point.
- Consider finding a **perinatal mental health certified (PMH-C)** therapist if you feel like you might benefit from processing your experience, even if it was decades ago. The **Postpartum Support International (PSI) HelpLine** is a great place to start.
- You don't owe anyone your story. Institutions are bigger drivers of stigma than individuals and whether or not they choose to share their trauma with others. But if sharing feels right for you, go for it. Storytelling is a powerful way of decreasing shame and stigma and encouraging others to get help.
- Check out books and podcasts related to maternal mental health, if hearing other stories like yours would be validating and/or comforting to you. There's a list of great podcasts, books, and films in the Appendix.

If you're pregnant or postpartum, or if you plan on having kids in the future...

- Add the **Health Resources and Services Administration (HRSA) Maternal Mental Health Hotline (1-833-TLC-MAMA)** to your contacts, and share it with your playgroup friends, mom group friends, high school friends, etc.

- Bookmark **Postpartum Support International (PSI)**, the largest maternal mental health advocacy organization, on your computer. They have all sorts of amazing resources, including free online support groups.

- Talk to your partner about maternal mental health conditions, and encourage them to learn about signs and symptoms so that they can help keep an eye on you throughout your journey.

- Consider finding a **perinatal mental health certified (PMH-C)** therapist if you need help. The **PSI HelpLine** is a great place to start.

- Create a postpartum plan, in the same way that you might make a birth plan. This can include identifying support people and strategizing about how to get uninterrupted blocks of sleep, how to ensure that you're getting adequate nutrition, etc. There are templates out there that you could use for more ideas.

- Check out podcasts related to maternal mental health, if podcasts are your thing. There's a list of great podcasts in the Appendix.

If you're the partner to someone who is, was, or plans to be pregnant...

- Learn about the wide range of signs and symptoms of maternal mental health conditions so that you can keep a close eye on your partner throughout their pregnancy and postpartum journey.

- Bookmark **Postpartum Support International (PSI)**, the largest maternal mental health advocacy organization. They have all sorts of amazing resources, including free online support groups (for you *and* for your partner).
- Do the legwork of helping your partner find an in-network, **perinatal mental health (PMH-C)**-trained mental health provider if needed. The **PSI HelpLine** is a great place to start.
- If you have paternity leave, take it. If you don't have paternity leave, speak up in your workplace and with policymakers about the burden this places on your family, so that families behind you might have a different experience.
- Help your partner create a postpartum plan, in the same way that you might help them make a birth plan. This can include identifying support people and strategizing about how to get uninterrupted blocks of sleep, how to ensure that you're getting adequate nutrition, etc. There are templates out there that you could use for more ideas.

If you're a general community member…
- Take additional training on recognizing the signs and symptoms of maternal mental health conditions and tips on how to respond if you encounter someone in need of help.
- Pay attention to and check in on any new moms in your life (friends, family members, coworkers, etc.), and offer tangible support if you can, such as meals, cleaning help, babysitting older children, etc.

- Learn about **Postpartum Support International (PSI)**, the largest maternal mental health advocacy organization. If and when you encounter someone in need of support, this is a good place to point them to. Consider supporting their work financially if you're in a position to do so.
- If nothing else, simply stop telling new moms to "enjoy every second" or to "just wait" for the challenging _______ stage. It helps no one, and it harms many.

If you're an OBGYN, midwife, psychiatrist, family medicine physician, emergency medicine physician, or pediatrician…

- Learn about **Postpartum Support International (PSI)**, the largest maternal mental health advocacy organization. If and when you encounter someone in need of support, this is a good place to point them to.
- Consider becoming **perinatal mental health certified (PMH-C)** if this is a topic you'd like to learn more about. At minimum, learn more about the ways in which maternal mental health conditions can present. They show up in ways other than excessive crying. Continue to normalize challenging experiences and feelings, but try to resist normalizing things that are actually signs or symptoms of a bigger problem.
- Learn whether or not your state has a **Perinatal Psychiatry Access Program** that provides free perinatal psychiatry consultations for prescribers treating perinatal patients. If it doesn't, **PSI** has a **Provider Psychiatric Consultation line** for prescribers that you could use if you need additional guidance when working with a perinatal patient.

- Reach out to your former training program to ask what kind of training they offer about maternal mental health conditions, and point them to resources (such as the **National Curriculum in Reproductive Psychiatry**) as needed. Including this topic in medical education is one of the highest-impact changes we could make.

- Resist the urge to see maternal mental health as "someone else's problem." This doesn't require you to become an expert in perinatal psychiatric care; you just need a basic awareness of how to respond empathetically and direct a patient toward someone who can help.

- Ask your health system, or health systems in your area, to implement evidence-based processes and build evidence-based programs to serve new parents. Let them know what you need in order to better care for this population.

- Learn about what, if any, perinatal intensive treatment options exist in your area. **PSI** has an **Intensive Treatment List** by state on their website, and I've built a tool where you can search by zip code for the nearest program that you can access via my **Mission Just One Mom** website (www.missionjustonemom.com). If and when you encounter a new mom in distress, let her know about the specific resource(s) in your area, if there are any. Remember that sifting through options is hard, if not impossible, when you're struggling.

If you're another kind of physician, NP, PA, or RN…

- Learn more about the ways in which maternal mental health conditions can present. They show up in ways other than excessive crying. Continue to normalize challenging experiences and feelings, but try to resist normalizing things that are actually signs or symptoms of a bigger problem.

- Reach out to your former training program to ask what kind of training they offer about maternal mental health conditions, and point them to resources (such as the **National Curriculum in Reproductive Psychiatry**) as needed.
- Resist the urge to see maternal mental health as "someone else's problem." This doesn't require you to become an expert in perinatal psychiatric care; you just need a basic awareness of how to respond empathetically and direct them toward someone who can help.
  - Even if you're a pediatric ophthalmologist, you may have an opportunity to intervene if you see warning signs of someone in distress.
- Ask your health system, or health systems in your area, to implement evidence-based processes and build evidence-based programs to serve new parents. Even if this is technically outside of your wheelhouse, your voice has an impact.
- Learn about **Postpartum Support International (PSI)**, the largest maternal mental health advocacy organization. If and when you encounter someone in need of support, this is a good place to point them to.

If you're any other type of birth worker (doula, lactation consultant, etc.)...
- Learn more about the ways in which maternal mental health conditions can present. They show up in ways other than excessive crying. Continue to normalize challenging experiences and feelings, but try to resist normalizing things that are actually signs or symptoms of a bigger problem.

- Learn about **Postpartum Support International (PSI)**, the largest maternal mental health advocacy organization. If and when you encounter someone in need of support, this is a good place to point them to.
- Reach out to your former training program to ask what kind of training they offer about maternal mental health conditions, and point them to resources (such as **PSI**) as needed.
- Ask your health system, or health systems in your area, to implement evidence-based processes and build evidence-based programs to serve new parents. Even if this is technically outside of your wheelhouse, your voice has an impact.

If you're a therapist or social worker...

- Learn about **Postpartum Support International (PSI)**, the largest maternal mental health advocacy organization. If and when you encounter someone in need of support, this is a good place to point them to.
- Consider becoming **perinatal mental health certified (PMH-C)** if this is a topic you'd like to learn more about.
- If you don't opt for additional training, refrain from promoting yourself as an expert in caring for pregnant or postpartum individuals. Lived experience or prior experience working with the perinatal population doesn't necessarily equate to clinical expertise in this subject, and the stakes are high.
- If you *are* PMH-C certified, sign up to be listed in the **PSI Provider Directory** so patients can find you more easily.

If you work in medical education...

- Incorporate information from the **National Curriculum in Reproductive Psychiatry** into your curriculum. I know your students have a lot to learn; I know adding new content means removing old content. But maternal mental health conditions affect 800,000+ people each year. It's the leading cause of maternal death. Find a way to add it.

If you're a payer…

- Review your reimbursement rates for perinatal mental health services, and ensure that providers are being offered fair and sustainable rates.

- Eliminate prior authorization requirements for perinatal mental health services. By definition, a request for perinatal mental health services implies that someone in distress is responsible for the well-being of an infant; there's no time to wait. It's highly unlikely that seeking additional mental health support is the wrong answer, and a very high chance that it's the right or even the life-saving answer.

- Assess network adequacy for perinatal mental health providers. Ensure members have access to **PMH-C**-certified therapists within a reasonable distance and time frame. Yes, I know that will require some manual work, because PMH-C is not a distinct type of professional with its own taxonomy (though perhaps it should be). Yes, you should still do it.

- Have a quality improvement team evaluate your current processes to determine whether you're currently meeting best practices and, if not, where your gaps lie and how you can remedy them. **The Policy Center for Maternal Mental Health** has a great resource you could use called the **Whole Mom Standards checklist.**

If you're a policymaker…

- Assess what policies and resources do and do not exist under your jurisdiction. The **Maternal Mental Health Leadership Alliance (MMHLA)** has resources by state for all 50 states plus D.C. and Puerto Rico.

- Learn whether or not your state has a **Perinatal Psychiatry Access Program**. If not, raise the question and do your research to determine if this is worth pursuing.

- Assess treatment resource gaps in your area using **The Policy Center for Maternal Mental Health's U.S. Maternal Mental Health Risk and Resources Maps**.

- Consult experts in maternal mental health, including those with lived experience, to better understand how existing and potential policies may help or hurt the well-being of new parents.

- Review the **National Strategy to Improve Maternal Mental Health**, published in 2024, for additional ideas and guidance.

If you're a journalist…

- As discussed, stop publishing postpartum psychosis click-bait. This is harmful on so many levels and demonstrates profound ignorance about maternal mental health.

- Educate your colleagues about this issue, and encourage them to re-think headlines that villainize moms with serious psychiatric conditions (or anyone with serious psychiatric conditions, for that matter). The **Maternal Mental Health Leadership Alliance (MMHLA)** has helpful, digestible fact sheets that you could share.

And finally, if you're a healthcare leader...

- Be humble. Be willing to admit that gaps exist. Be willing to admit that those gaps have allowed harm to occur. Be willing to admit that those gaps have probably *caused* harm. Looking directly at the gaps is the way to close them and move forward.

- Ensure that all providers who regularly interact with your perinatal patients have a baseline competence in maternal mental health. This includes anyone working in primary care, women's health, pediatrics, urgent care, mental health, or the ER. **Postpartum Support International (PSI)** offers several levels of provider training.

- Survey all of your ERs. Ensure that they have the necessary supplies to accommodate women with infants, including bassinets and pumps. Mothers in crisis (physical or mental) shouldn't have to choose between getting help and caring for their infant. Remember that not every woman has a village to lean on in emergency situations.

- Determine who has ultimate responsibility for maternal mental health processes and outcomes at your organization. The answer is not "women's health and behavioral health." Pick someone to hold the responsibility, or create a new position for this purpose. Everyone's responsibility is nobody's responsibility.

- Assess your perinatal mental health screening process. The most comprehensive information and guidance on this can be found in the **UMass Chan Lifeline for Moms Toolkit**. You can find more information about this resource on the **American College of Obstetricians and Gynecologists** website as well.

- Have a quality improvement team evaluate your current processes to determine whether you're currently meeting best practices and, if not, where your gaps lie and how you can remedy them. **The Policy Center for Maternal Mental Health** has a great resource you can use called the **Whole Mom Standards checklist**.
- Ask your OBGYNs, L&D RNs, psychiatrists, pediatricians, etc. what else you can do to make it easier for them to provide high-quality care to pregnant and postpartum people. Act upon their feedback.
- Check in on your physicians who are also mothers. Physician mothers are at increased risk for maternal mental health conditions. Remember that the medical system was built when most doctors were men with wives at home. That world doesn't exist anymore. Now, over half of medical school graduates are women, and many are or will become moms at some point in their career. Implement family-friendly policies like on-site lactation spaces, flexible scheduling for parents, and backup childcare options.
- Ask your patients for feedback, and listen with an open mind. Include patient representatives in the quality improvement process. Remember what I said (and you first taught me) about the Swiss cheese model? Patients with lived experience are the ones who can most reliably show you where the holes are.

Everyone...
- There are a lot of big problems in the world that can seem, at times, like a lost cause. Fight the urge to consider maternal mental health one of them. Your actions

matter, and you have the power to potentially change the narrative, even if just slightly, for another family.

- Be kind.

This list isn't perfect. But it's a start. And I guarantee that if everyone reading this book implements even one of the suggestions listed, the world will be a friendlier place for new mothers.

Concluding With Gratitude

I want to close out this book where my advocacy efforts all started: with profound gratitude.

Everything I say and everything I do on this topic stems from gratitude that I got to fully recover from something that has ruthlessly stolen the lives of so many. Diving into advocacy has forced me well outside of my comfort zone, but I do it because I'm so thankful I get to be alive today to enjoy the heck out of my son. I hope that's evident, no matter how punchy or provocative my words are. At the end of the day, it's all because I feel like I won the lottery, and this is my honest effort to pay it forward and bend the trajectory for those behind me.

Thank you to anyone who took the time to read this book, who had an interest in learning more about maternal mental health disorders and how we can collectively do more to reduce their impact on individuals and on our society (especially those who are now teeming with frustration and determined to do something with what they've learned).

Thank you to everyone who's already actively doing something to improve the state of maternal mental health, whether as a clinician, a therapist, a nonprofit leader, a community volunteer, or simply as a caring friend or family member. Along the way, during my illness as well as during my recovery, I've met some truly incredible human beings who are deeply committed to helping others navigate maternal mental health issues. To use a cliché, this is the coolest club I never wanted to be a part of.

And finally, thank you to all the women and families who've walked this road before me, who bravely shared their trauma with the world in the name of saving the next woman from the same experience. By advocating for awareness, resources, and specialized programs, you saved my life. The only way I know to adequately thank you is to pay it forward by adding my story to the pile and my voice to the fight.

I want to close by posing a question to Leader C, in case you're reading this: just to confirm, am I too close to this topic to be a useful participant in the conversation, or am I just close enough?

Epilogue

It's February of 2026, and for the second time, I'm nine weeks and one day pregnant.

In some ways, my experience so far has been similar to the last, because once again, I'm more than three weeks into something that it's fair to describe as a "24/7 nausea hellscape." But in other ways, this pregnancy has already been much different. Instead of suffering in silence, I chose to share the news with my family and close friends much sooner, so that it would be easier to request and receive support (both physical and emotional). I've also been more assertive with my care team about exactly how awful I'm feeling, and as a result, I've been offered more treatment options to try.

My maternal mental health recovery and advocacy journey taught me many things, among them that advocating for yourself matters. The default setting of our healthcare system, nationally, is to downplay and dismiss women's discomfort. That's not a knock on current providers, who are typically doing their best to provide the highest-quality care they can. It's merely a statement on our underlying women's health infrastructure, which is overdue for a significant upgrade (as I hope you now agree).

Another thing that has been different so far is the level of anxiety I feel about the pregnancy overall. While I know that anything can happen and nothing is guaranteed, I now have proof, in the form of my happy, healthy, goofy toddler, that my body *can* successfully carry and deliver a child. I also now have proof, in the form of my happy, healthy, goofy toddler, that I am capable of being a good mother. Those core fears that began to eat away at me during my first pregnancy are no longer riding shotgun this time around.

I'm often asked whether I'm scared to go down this road again after how painful and scary it was last time. The answer is yes, without question. But what grounds me, and, frankly, what allowed me to make this choice again, was knowing that my experience cannot be the same. I could have similar challenges with unrelenting nausea (check), and later down the road I could have similar challenges with delivery. I could even face some of the same scary mental health symptoms during pregnancy and/or the postpartum period.

But even if that all happens, which I hope it doesn't, the circumstances surrounding those things would be different. I'm on medication, I have an ongoing relationship with a therapist, and I have experience navigating the behavioral system, all of which I didn't have before. And perhaps most importantly, I now have vocabulary to describe the symptoms I might experience and knowledge of where to turn if things get hard. There's no scenario in which I find myself in the position I was nearly three years ago, when I had no knowledge of potential postpartum mental health complications beyond depression and therefore assumed I was suffering from something rare and untreatable.

So yes, I'm terrified, but yes, I'm doing it anyway. Alex and I have talked about wanting to have kids, plural, since our earliest days together, and that desire hasn't changed despite everything we've gone through. So, I'm holding hope alongside my fears, and gratitude for this pregnancy alongside my discomfort.

Thank you to everyone who's read this far, and to everyone who's supporting me both in my advocacy journey and on my road to becoming a second-time mom. I hope this book has helped you feel less alone, more equipped to demand better from our healthcare system, or both.

Em

Acknowledgments

First and foremost, I'd like to thank every single woman who came before me and spoke up about her journey with a maternal mental health condition, thus decreasing the stigma around it and paving the way to the resources I ultimately had access to. I don't for a second believe I would've been brave enough to speak so openly about this topic if this experience had happened to me 20+ years earlier. Your stories have saved lives and opened the door for others to share their most vulnerable experiences, too. On a similar note, thank you to Steven D'Achille and his daughter Adrianna, for turning pain into purpose and saving the lives of so many women through the Alexis Joy Center.

Next, I'd like to thank the team of professionals who helped me bring the final product of this book to life. Thank you to my copy editor Claire Dunn for being so thorough, quick, and compassionate. Thank you to my designer Danna Steele for creating both a beautiful cover and a beautiful interior, and thank you to Maria Sosnowski for making it easier for others to use this book by creating a detailed index.

Thank you to "Dr. E," for founding the partial hospitalization program I attended, for providing me and my family with our first glimmer of hope, and for helping me understand how uniquely bad the U.S. is at supporting new parents relative to the rest of the world. Thank you to Taylor Garmaker, CPD, CLS for walking alongside me in the darkness as a peer support mentor, and to my "Mental Health Besties" SZ, SR, and KT, for continuing the group therapy off-line, for inspiring and encouraging me to fight this fight, and for always being there to celebrate both the highs and the lows of early parenthood. Thank you to my therapist, for helping me evolve from a woman who was functional but still terrified to face her story to a woman who is confident telling and re-telling her story, warts and all.

Thank you to Matthew Holt for giving me a platform to share my story in writing for the first time, and to Joy Burkhard, MBA for giving me a platform to publicly share my story out loud for the first time and for being such a forceful advocate for new mothers in the U.S. I am so grateful for everything you've done to bring awareness to this issue and address the systemic issues that lie behind it all. And thank you to everyone else I have met in the maternal mental health advocacy world who is doing amazing work to support current and future mothers and families: you inspire me every single day.

Thank you to my MHA program professors for equipping me with the training and the confidence needed to face a problem like this head-on, and for supporting me as I began to raise my voice. Thank you to GH for being a sounding board regarding this enormous career pivot and for supporting my decision to chart a new path for myself. Thank you to my incredible former boss "Deb" for being supportive of me telling my story and of chasing my dream to help other moms and families. Your leadership left an impression on me that I carry with me today.

And finally, thank you to my friends and family. Starting with my own mom, who fought like hell to find me help and wouldn't accept no for an answer, joined me in this discovery journey about maternal mental health care, and supported every single piece of this book project. Thank you to Melissa Hibdon, RN, MBA, and more importantly, my aunt, for taking charge when I needed it most and for jumping into the pit with me, no questions asked. Thank you to Sarah Schahrer, for walking in when others walked out, holding my grief with me, and somehow also making me laugh. Thank you to Maya Sorini, MD for encouraging me to dream big and fight like hell for future patients. Thank you to my dad, my siblings, and all my in-laws for supporting me in this passion project and for being part of my village in raising Julian. Thank you to all the amazing kids in my life who remind me of who I'm fighting for, including my son Julian, my nieces and nephews, and the dozens upon dozens of hard-working gymnasts I coach. And last but not least, thank you to my husband Alex, who never wavered in his support for me, both during the postpartum period and when I ultimately left my job and began my advocacy work to start putting our shared trauma on display. I love you more than anything, and I'm so thankful for our life together.

Appendix

A SURVIVOR'S GUIDE TO PERINATAL MENTAL HEALTH RESOURCES

There are some absolutely incredible individuals and organizations out there putting in the work to ensure that moms and families in the U.S. have access to the support they need to thrive. There are also several books, podcasts, and films that help explain and illuminate the issue, as well as training opportunities for those who want to explore this topic further.

Most near and dear to my heart, there are also several programs out there offering intensive treatment to perinatal women, similar to the one I had the opportunity to attend. I've listed them all here, and I encourage you to support these programs and/or refer others to them as appropriate.

Part I: Organizations Related to Maternal Mental Health
Part II: Books, Podcasts, and Films About Maternal Mental Health
Part III: Training Opportunities
Part IV: Intensive Treatment Programs in the United States

ORGANIZATIONS RELATED TO MATERNAL MENTAL HEALTH

Below, you'll find some of the organizations I've learned about or worked with in my advocacy journey so far. This list is *not* an exhaustive list of all organizations contributing to the field; rather, it features organizations I've come across as a survivor and a patient advocate. This list is United States-centric given the scope of my experience and, subsequently, this book.

Organization	Year Est.	Topic
The Marcé Society and The Marcé Society of North America (MONA)	1980	International, interdisciplinary organization dedicated to supporting research and assistance surrounding prenatal and postpartum mental health. The North American regional organization was created around 2015.
Postpartum Support International (PSI)	1987	Nonprofit organization that raises awareness of perinatal mental health disorders, offers training and resources for professionals, and helps people find and connect to appropriate treatment.

The Policy Center for Maternal Mental Health	2011	Nonprofit organization that brings together key stakeholders (payers, providers, policymakers) to drive tangible improvements in maternal mental healthcare at the system level.
The Alexis Joy Foundation	2013	Nonprofit organization founded in honor of Alexis D'Achille that led to the development of an intensive outpatient program for perinatal women in Pittsburgh, PA.
Shades of Blue Project	2013	Survivor-led nonprofit organization focused on improving maternal mental health outcomes for black and brown birthing people.
National Birth Equity Collaborative	2015	Nonprofit working to improve rates of infant mortality and maternal mortality within Black and Brown communities through training, research, technical assistance, policy, advocacy, and community-centered collaboration.
Black Mamas Matter Alliance	2016	Nonprofit that advocates for birth and reproductive justice for Black mothers. They host Black Maternal Health Week as well as an annual conference.
Cherished Mom	2018	Survivor-led advocacy group focusing on pregnancy and postpartum psychosis and the prevention of maternal suicide.
MoMMAs Voices	2018	Nonprofit organization that empowers and equips moms to tell their maternal health stories and helps healthcare organizations find individuals with lived experience to inform improvement efforts.

Maternal Mental Health Leadership Alliance	2019	Nonprofit advocacy organization focused on driving legislative changes to improve maternal mental health.
Perinatal Quality Collaboratives	Varies by state	Organizations that lead and coordinate maternal health quality improvement efforts.
Chamber of Mothers	2021	Bipartisan nonprofit organization that brings moms together to advance maternal rights in the U.S.
The Dr. Mom Foundation	2021	Advocacy related to the intersection between maternal mental health and women in medicine (an at-risk group for postpartum depression).

While not an independent organization, **Maternal Mortality Review Committees (MMRCs)** are another vital contributor to maternal mental awareness and improvement. These are state-based multidisciplinary committees that comprehensively review deaths that occur during or within one year of the end of pregnancy. While some forms of MMRCs have been around since the 1930s, they were federally funded by the Preventing Maternal Deaths Act of 2018.

PART II

BOOKS, PODCASTS, AND FILMS ABOUT MATERNAL MENTAL HEALTH

Here are a few great books, podcasts, and films I recommend checking out if you're interested in learning more about maternal mental health and what these experiences look and feel like for women and their families. I remember it being difficult to find these kinds of resources when I was struggling, so here's a starting point. This is by no means an exhaustive list, just ones I'm familiar with.

Books

Book Title	Author	Pub. Year(s)*
This Isn't What I Expected: Overcoming Postpartum Depression	Karen Kleiman, MSW, LCSW	1994, 2025
Good Moms Have Scary Thoughts: A Healing Guide to the Secret Fears of New Mothers	Karen Kleiman, MSW, LCSW	2019

Down Came The Rain: My Journey Through Postpartum Depression	Brooke Shields	2005
Beyond the Blues: A Guide to Understanding and Treating Prenatal And Postpartum Depression	Shoshana Bennett, PhD and Pec Indman, EdD, MFT	2006, 2024
Day Nine: A Postpartum Depression Memoir	Amanda Munday	2019
Motherhood and Mental Illness: A Relational Treatment Approach	Emma Hayes	2022
Blue: A History of Postpartum Depression in America	Rachel Moran, PhD	2024
A Mom Like That: A Memoir of Postpartum Psychosis	Aaisha Alvi	2024
Then Comes Baby: An Honest Conversation about Birth, Postpartum, and the Complex Transition to Parenthood	Jessica Vernon, MD	2025

*Books with multiple editions list first and last years of publication only

Podcasts

Title	Host	Topic/Niche
PSI I am One	Postpartum Support International	Stories from people with lived experience
Mom and Mind	Katayune Kaeni, Psy.D, PMH-C	Everything about maternal mental health
The Mama Making Podcast	Jessica Lamb	Expert interviews and stories about motherhood, not limited to mental health disorders
Healing the Tigress	Peggy (LCSW, PMH-C) and Jasmine (PharmD, PMH-C)	Conversation and stories around Asian American Pacific Islander (AAPI) maternal mental health stories

All the Hard Things	Jenna Overbaugh, LPC	OCD stories and tips
Mom Breaks	Meg, PPP survivor	Postpartum psychosis stories
More than Mom	Dr. Nichelle Haynes, MD, perinatal psychiatrist	Conversations about mental health and motherhood led by an expert in perinatal psychiatry
Is Mom Okay?	Cherished Mom	Postpartum psychosis stories

Films

24 Days Without You is a documentary produced by Rebecca Rizio and Annie Sterle, an amniotic fluid embolism survivor. It was released in 2024 and covers her experience with significant birth complications, as well as the psychological aftermath of that devastating experience.

More Than Blue is a documentary produced by Lee Cohen, MD, also released in 2024.

You're Not Alone: Pregnancy, Postpartum and the Mental Health Crisis is a short documentary published in 2023 by WQED Pittsburgh. It's publicly available on YouTube.

PART III

MATERNAL MENTAL HEALTH TRAINING OPPORTUNITIES

Below, you'll find a guide to organizations that offer training on perinatal mental health. This isn't an exhaustive list, just a starting point you can use to begin your research.

The **Maternal Mental Health Leadership Alliance** has a searchable online database of maternal mental health training courses, which enables you to search by topic, profession, length, and other criteria. This database includes the courses offered by the organizations highlighted below.

Third-Party Organizations

Courses offered by any of these nonprofit organizations can be taken by healthcare professionals. Many of them can also be taken by anyone and everyone who wants to learn more about maternal mental health disorders and how to support new moms.

Postpartum Support International offers several different types of training, including a two-and-a-half-day course that prepares professionals to take the PMH-C certification exam, specialized perinatal loss training, specialized paternal mental health training, and more.

The Policy Center for Maternal Mental Health offers both comprehensive certificate training courses and free online webinars on a variety of topics related to maternal mental health.

The Seleni Institute offers several expert-led, evidence-based training courses in reproductive and maternal mental health, including topics like adolescent perinatal mental health and Black perinatal mental health.

For physicians and other mental health professionals, the **National Curriculum in Reproductive Psychiatry** offers online and in-person opportunities to improve your knowledge of the diagnosis and treatment of psychiatric disorders throughout the reproductive life span.

Medical Training Programs

For **psychiatrists** looking to become experts in reproductive psychiatry, there are currently 16 reproductive psychiatry fellowships in the U.S. They are located in:

- Illinois (3)
- Massachusetts (2)
- Maryland
- New Mexico
- New York (4)
- North Carolina
- Ohio

- Rhode Island
- South Carolina
- Washington

There's also one in Toronto, Canada.

The Marcé Society of North America maintains a list of these programs, which can be found at marcenortham.com/fellowships

PART IV

INTENSIVE TREATMENT PROGRAMS IN THE UNITED STATES

Below, you'll find a list of perinatal intensive treatment programs in the United States by level of care. My mom, the incredible and thorough Ginna Ericksen, has personally called to verify the existence of each of these programs, so this should be a fairly accurate list as of early 2026.

She also volunteers with Postpartum Support International to help maintain the intensive treatment program information on their website.[81] For the most up-to-date information, I recommend checking their list. Kudos to all of the programs on this list: you've rolled a boulder uphill to provide specialized care for the new moms in your community, and your work matters. A lot.

Perinatal Intensive Outpatient Programs (IOPs) in the U.S.

Name	City	State	Year Est.
El Camino Hospital Maternal Outreach Mood Services (MOMS)	Mountain View	CA	2008
Ascension Illinois Perinatal IOP at Saint Alexius Women & Children's Hospital	Hoffman Estates	IL	2015
Alexis Joy D'Achille Center for Women's Behavioral Health at West Penn Hospital	Pittsburgh	PA	2015
Drexel University Mother Baby Connections IOP	*Virtual Only*	PA	2015
Serenity Recovery and Wellness	Riverton	UT	2017
Reach Counseling Utah.com	*Virtual Only*	UT	2017
UCLA CA Resnick/Maternal Mental Health Program	Los Angeles	CA	2017
Sagent (Formerly Nystrom & Associate's) Mother Baby	Baxter, Eden Prairie, Otsego, St. Cloud	MN	2017
Sagent (Formerly Nystrom & Associate's) Mother Baby	Fargo	ND	2017
PrairieCare Mother-Baby IOP	*Virtual Only*	MN	2019
Serenity Recovery and Wellness	Provo	UT	2019
Providence Mission Hospital	*Virtual Only*	CA	2020
Anchor Perinatal Wellness IOP	Raleigh	NC	2022
Macari Perinatal Intensive Outpatient Program	Forest Hills	NY	2022
Mercy Birthplace Mother-Baby Intensive Outpatient Program	St. Louis	MO	2022
River Root Counseling Mother & Baby Perinatal IOP	*Virtual Only*	OH	2022
UPMC Magee Women's Perinatal OCD & Anxiety IOP	*Virtual Only*	PA	2022

The Motherhood Space Day Program	Jacksonville	FL	2023
Sharp Mesa Vista - Maternal Mental Health IOP	San Diego	CA	2024
Sutter Center for Psychiatry Perinatal IOP	*Virtual Only*	CA	2024
Healthy Expectations Perinatal Intensive Outpatient Program	Aurora	CO	2024
Allied Behavioral Health Solutions: Rooted Connections Perinatal Mental Health	*Virtual Only*	TN	2024
Henrico Doctors Hospital Women's Perinatal & Postpartum Mental Health Program	Richmond	VA	2024
MedStar Health Mother-Baby Intensive Outpatient Program	Washington DC	DC	2024
University Hospitals Perinatal Behavioral Health Services, Cleveland	*Virtual Only*	OH	2024
Perinatal Day Program at the Institute of Living	Hartford	CT	2025
Tulia Grove	Live Oak	TX	2025
The Bloom Center	*Virtual Only*	TX	2025
The Postpartum Den	Nashville	TN	2025
Prisma Health Mother-Infant Wellness Program	Greenville	SC	2025
Root + Rise Perinatal	Rockland	MA	2025
Soleo Wellness	Duxbury	MA	2025
Inner Community Health	Duluth	GA	2025
Mindful Health: Mindful Maternity Perinatal IOP	*Virtual Only*	TX	2026
Huntington Memorial Hospital Maternal Wellness Program	*Virtual Only*	CA	Unknown
Women & Infants Hospital of RI Perinatal OCD IOP	Providence	RI	Unknown

Perinatal Partial Hospitalization Programs (PHPs)

Name	City	State	Year Est.
Brown/Women & Infants Day Hospital Program	Providence	RI	2000
El Camino Hospital Maternal Outreach Mood Services	Mountain View	CA	2008
Pine Rest Mother and Baby Program (Faith-based—Christian)	Grand Rapids	MI	2012
Redleaf Center for Family Healing Mother-Baby PHP	Minneapolis	MN	2013
Swedish Perinatal Center for Perinatal Bonding and Support	Seattle	WA	2016
The Motherhood Center of New York	New York City	NY	2017
Mother-Infant Wellness Program	Greenville	SC	2025
Soleo Wellness	Duxbury	MA	2025

Perinatal Inpatient Units in the United States

Hospital/Program	City	State	Year Est.	Beds
UNC Center for Women's Mood Disorders	Chapel Hill	NC	2011	5
UAMS Psychiatry Research Institute	Little Rock	AR	2013	10
Northwell, Zucker Hillside Hospital	Glen Oaks	NY	2016	22
El Camino Hospital Women's Specialty Unit	Mountain View	CA	2020	6-9
Woman's Hospital	Baton Rouge	LA	2024	10

ENDNOTES

1   Clarke, D. E., De Faria, L., & Alpert, J.E, The Perinatal Mental Health
    Advisory Panel, The Perinatal Mental Health Research Team. (2023).
    Perinatal mental and substance use disorder [White paper]. American
    Psychiatric Association. Available from https://www.psychiatry.org/maternal

2   Centers for Disease Control and Prevention. (2025, August 22). *Pregnancy-
    related deaths: Data from Maternal Mortality Review Committees.* https://
    www.cdc.gov/maternal-mortality/php/data-research/mmrc-2017-2019.html

3   Maternal Mental Health Leadership Alliance. (2024, October 10). *Maternal
    mental health conditions and statistics: An overview.* https://www.mmhla.org/
    articles/maternal-mental-health-conditions-and-statistics

4   Tauri, N., & Duerr, H. E. (2023, June 2). Multidisciplinary program
    improves perinatal depressive symptoms. *Psychiatric Times.* https://www.
    psychiatrictimes.com/view/multidisciplinary-program-improves-perinatal-
    depressive-symptoms

5   Howard, M., Battle, C. L., Pearlstein, T., & Rosene-Montella, K. (2006). A
    psychiatric mother-baby day hospital for pregnant and postpartum women.
    Archives of Women's Mental Health, 9(4), 213–218. https://doi.org/10.1007/
    s00737-006-0135-y

6   Levinson, Z., Godwin, G., & Neuman, T. (2024, December 18). *Hospital
    margins rebounded in 2023, but rural hospitals and those with High Medicaid
    shares were struggling more than others.* KFF. https://www.kff.org/health-costs/
    hospital-margins-rebounded-in-2023-but-rural-hospitals-and-those-with-
    high-medicaid-shares-were-struggling-more-than-others/

7   Torrance, L. (2018, December 18). AHN Opens Alexis Joy D'Achille
    Center for postpartum depression. *Pittsburgh Business Times.* https://www.
    bizjournals.com/pittsburgh/news/2018/12/18/ahn-opens-alexis-joy-dachille-
    center-for.html

8   Birk, S. (n.d.). *The promise and practice of a just culture.* Healthcare
    Executive. https://healthcareexecutive.org/archives/march-april-2020/the-
    promise-and-practice-of-a-just-culture

9   Grigoriadis, S., Graves, L., Peer, M., Mamisashvili, L., Tomlinson, G.,
    Vigod, S. N., Dennis, C. L., Steiner, M., Brown, C., Cheung, A., Dawson,
    H., Rector, N. A., Guenette, M., & Richter, M. (2018). Maternal anxiety

during pregnancy and the association with adverse perinatal outcomes: Systematic review and meta-analysis. *The Journal of Clinical Psychiatry*, *79*(5), 17r12011. https://doi.org/10.4088/JCP.17r12011

10 Gruszczyńska-Sińczak, I., Wachowska, K., Bliźniewska-Kowalska, K., & Gałecki, P. (2023). Psychiatric treatment in pregnancy: A narrative review. *Journal of Clinical Medicine*, *12*(14), 4746. https://doi.org/10.3390/jcm12144746.

11 Wiginton, K. (n.d.). *What are intrusive thoughts?* WebMD. https://www.webmd.com/mental-health/intrusive-thoughts

12 International OCD Foundation. (n.d.). *Perinatal OCD overview.* https://iocdf.org/perinatal-ocd/for-clinical-providers/perinatal-ocd-overview/

13 National Academies of Sciences, Engineering, and Medicine; Health and Medicine Division; Board on Population Health and Public Health Practice; Committee on Applying Neurobiological and Socio-Behavioral Sciences from Prenatal Through Early Childhood Development: A Health Equity Approach, Negussie, Y., Geller, A., & DeVoe, J. E. (Eds.). (2019). *Vibrant and healthy kids: Aligning science, practice, and policy to advance health equity.* National Academies Press (US). https://doi.org/10.17226/25466

14 NHS. (n.d.). *Symptoms – postnatal depression.* https://www.nhs.uk/mental-health/conditions/post-natal-depression/symptoms

15 Pawlowski, A. (2019, May 20). *Car seat danger: Babies shouldn't sleep in car seats when not traveling.* Today. https://www.today.com/health/car-seat-danger-babies-shouldn-t-sleep-car-seats-when-t154353

16 Postpartum Support International. (n.d.). *Perinatal mental health: Signs, symptoms and treatment.* https://postpartum.net/perinatal-mental-health/

17 Jana , L. A., & Shu, J. (2024, July 11). *Pooping by the numbers: What's normal for infants?* HealthyChildren.org. https://www.healthychildren.org/English/ages-stages/baby/Pages/Pooping-By-the-Numbers.aspx

18 Cornett, E. M., Rando, L., Labbé, A. M., Perkins, W., Kaye, A. M., Kaye, A. D., Viswanath, O., & Urits, I. (2021). Brexanolone to treat postpartum depression in adult women. *Psychopharmacology Bulletin*, *51*(2), 115–130. https://doi.org/10.64719/pb.4397

19 Cornett, E. M., Rando, L., Labbé, A. M., Perkins, W., Kaye, A. M., Kaye, A. D., Viswanath, O., & Urits, I. (2021). Brexanolone to treat postpartum depression in adult women. Psychopharmacology Bulletin, 51(2), 115–130. https://doi.org/10.64719/pb.4397

20 Bodenheimer, T., & Sinsky, C. (2014). From triple to quadruple aim: Care of the patient requires care of the provider. *Annals of Family Medicine*, *12*(6), 573–576. https://doi.org/10.1370/afm.1713

21 MacMillan, C. (2023, September 15). What to know about Zurzuvae, the new pill to treat postpartum depression. Yale Medicine. https://www.yalemedicine.org/news/postpartum-depression-pill-zurzuvae-zuranolone

22 CBS News. (2023, September 15). *A promising treatment for postpartum depression* [Video]. https://www.cbsnews.com/video/a-promising-treatment-for-postpartum-depression/

23 Centers for Disease Control and Prevention. (n.d.). *HEAR HER campaign.* https://www.cdc.gov/hearher/index.html

24 Kachalia, A., Kaufman, S. R., Boothman, R., Anderson, S., Welch, K., Saint, S., & Rogers, M. A. (2010). Liability claims and costs before and after implementation of a medical error disclosure program. *Annals of Internal Medicine*, 153(4), 213–221. https://doi.org/10.7326/0003-4819-153-4-201008170-00002

25 Gavin, K. (2016, May 23). *Hospitals can break through the 'wall of silence' with new toolkit.* Michigan Medicine, University of Michigan. https://www.michiganmedicine.org/health-lab/hospitals-can-break-through-wall-silence-new-toolkit

26 Gavin, K. (2016, May 23). *Hospitals can break through the 'wall of silence' with new toolkit.* Michigan Medicine, University of Michigan. https://www.michiganmedicine.org/health-lab/hospitals-can-break-through-wall-silence-new-toolkit

27 National Center for Health Statistics. (n.d.). *Child health.* Centers for Disease Control and Prevention. https://www.cdc.gov/nchs/fastats/child-health.htm

28 Shepherd-Banigan, M., & Bell, J. F. (2014). Paid leave benefits among a national sample of working mothers with infants in the United States. *Maternal and Child Health Journal*, 18(1), 286–295. https://doi.org/10.1007/s10995-013-1264-3

29 *Postnatal rituals from around the world.* (2023, April 24). The Mindful Birth Group. https://www.themindfulbirthgroup.com/parents/blog/postnatal-rituals-from-around-the-world/

30 Osborne, L. M., Hermann, A., Burt, V., Driscoll, K., Fitelson, E., Meltzer-Brody, S., Barzilay, E. M., Yang, S. N., Miller, L., & National Task Force on Women's Reproductive Mental Health (2015). Reproductive psychiatry: The gap between clinical need and education. *The American Journal of Psychiatry*, 172(10), 946–948. https://doi.org/10.1176/appi.ajp.2015.15060837

31 Livingston, G. (2018, January 18). *They're waiting longer, but U.S. women today more likely to have children than a decade ago.* Pew Research Center. https://www.pewresearch.org/social-trends/2018/01/18/theyre-waiting-longer-but-u-s-women-today-more-likely-to-have-children-than-a-decade-ago/

32 Sheikh, M. H., Chaudhary, A. M. D., Khan, A. S., Tahir, M. A., Yahya, H. A., Naveed, S., & Khosa, F. (2018). Influences for gender disparity in academic psychiatry in the United States. *Cureus, 10*(4), e2514. https://doi.org/10.7759/cureus.2514

33 McNally, S. T., Miller, J., Patel, V., Hy, J., Shrivastava, S., & Pekmekzaris, R. (2024). An obstetrics & gynecology resident education program to address gaps in the knowledge, screening, and treatment of postpartum mood and anxiety disorder (PMAD). *Journal of Gynecological & Obstetrical Research, 2*(1), 1–6.

34 Vernon, J. (2025, April 17). *What PSI means to me as an OB/GYN.* Postpartum Support International. https://postpartum.net/what-psi-means-to-me-as-an-ob-gy

35 Colina, C., & Pope, D. (2025). Antidepressant use before, during, and after pregnancy. *JAMA Network Open, 8*(1), e2457324. https://doi.org/10.1001/jamanetworkopen.2024.57324

36 Marcé of North America. (n.d.). *Fellowship programs.* https://marcenortham.com/fellowships

37 Richmond, L. M. (2022). Trainees form new reproductive psychiatry group to learn, network, collaborate. *Psychiatric News, 57*(3). https://doi.org/10.1176/appi.pn.2022.03.3.46

38 National Curriculum in Reproductive Psychiatry. (n.d.). *About the National Curriculum in Reproductive Psychiatry.* https://ncrptraining.org/about/

39 National Curriculum in Reproductive Psychiatry. (n.d.). *NCRP & MONA: A valued partnership.* https://ncrptraining.org/ncrp-mona/

40 Postpartum Support International. (n.d.). *Certification in perinatal mental health.* https://postpartum.net/professionals/certification/

41 Postpartum Support International. (n.d.). *Certification in perinatal mental health.* https://postpartum.net/professionals/certification/

42 American College of Obstetricians & Gynecologists. (n.d.). *Perinatal mental health.* https://www.acog.org/programs/perinatal-mental-health

43 Policy Center for Maternal Mental Health (2025, May 28). *2025 U.S. maternal mental health risks and resources by county.* https://policycentermmh.org/2025-us-maternal-mental-health-risk-and-resources/

44 Care New England Women and Children's Hospital. (n.d.). *The Day Hospital.* https://www.womenandinfants.org/the-day-hospital

45 Battle, C. L., & Howard, M. M. (2014). A mother-baby psychiatric day hospital: History, rationale, and why perinatal mental health is important for obstetric medicine. *Obstetric Medicine, 7*(2), 66–70. https://doi.org/10.1177/1753495X13514402

46   Kim, H. G., Erickson, N. L., & Flynn, J. M. (2021). Keeping parent, child, and relationship in mind: Clinical effectiveness of a trauma-informed, multigenerational, attachment-based, mother-baby partial hospital program in an urban safety net hospital. *Maternal and Child Health Journal, 25*(11), 1776–1786. https://doi.org/10.1007/s10995-021-03221-4

47   McCabe-Beane, J. E., Segre, L. S., Perkhounkova, Y., Stuart, S., & O'Hara, M. W. (2016). The identification of severity ranges for the Edinburgh Postnatal Depression Scale. *Journal of Reproductive and Infant Psychology, 34*(3), 293–303. https://doi.org/10.1080/02646838.2016.1141346

48   Anxiety & Depression Society of America. (n.d.). *GAD-7 anxiety.* https://adaa.org/sites/default/files/GAD-7_Anxiety-updated_0.pdf

49   Gelabert E, Torres Giménez A, Andrés-Perpiñá S, Naranjo C, Roda E, Garcia-Esteve L, Roca Lecumberri A. (2022). Mother-baby day hospital (MBDH): Preliminary results of effectiveness of multidisciplinary intensive intervention for women with postpartum affective/anxiety disorder. *European Psychiatry, 65*(Suppl 1), S331. https://doi.org/10.1192/j.eurpsy.2022.843

50   Perigee Fund. (n.d.). *Mother-baby programs preserve critical bonding period.* https://perigeefund.org/stories/mother-baby-programs-preserve-critical-bonding-period/

51   Dembosky, A. (2021). A humane approach to caring for new mothers in psychiatric crisis. *Health Affairs, 40*(10), 1528–1533. https://www.healthaffairs.org/doi/10.1377/hlthaff.2021.01288

52   Centers for Disease Control and Prevention. (2026, March 2). *About adverse childhood experiences.* https://www.cdc.gov/aces/about/index.html

53   Alford, A. Y., Riggins, A. D., Chopak-Foss, J., Cowan, L. T., Nwaonumah, E. C., Oloyede, T. F., Sejoro, S. T., & Kutten, W. S. (2025). A systematic review of postpartum psychosis resulting in infanticide: Missed opportunities in screening, diagnosis, and treatment. *Archives of Women's Mental Health, 28*(2), 297–308. https://doi.org/10.1007/s00737-024-01508-3

54   Meltzer-Brody, S., Brandon, A. R., Pearson, B., Burns, L., Raines, C., Bullard, E., & Rubinow, D. (2014). Evaluating the clinical effectiveness of a specialized perinatal psychiatry inpatient unit. *Archives of Women's Mental Health, 17*(2), 107–113. https://doi.org/10.1007/s00737-013-0390-7

55   Cleveland Clinic. (2022, September 13). *Postpartum psychosis.* https://my.clevelandclinic.org/health/diseases/24152-postpartum-psychosis

56   Postpartum Support International. (n.d.). *Intensive treatment in the US.* https://postpartum.net/get-help/intensive-perinatal-psych-treatment-in-the-us/

57   Royal College of Psychiatrists. (2021, September). *Perinatal mental health services: Recommendations for the provision of services for childbearing women.* www.rcpsych.ac.uk/improving-care/campaigning-for-better-mental-health-

policy/college-reports/2021-college-reports/perinatal-mental-health-services-CR232.

58   Maternal Mental Health Alliance. (n.d.). *Improving access to specialist services.* https://maternalmentalhealthalliance.org/campaign/improving-services/specialist-services/

59   *Woman's Hospital: Extending the reach of care with new inpatient perinatal mental health unit.* (2024, April 8). Business Report. https://www.businessreport.com/sponsored/whats-new-in-health-care/womans-hospital-extending-the-reach-of-care-with-new-inpatient-perinatal-mental-health-unit

60   Levinson, Z., Hulver, S., Godwin, J., & Neuman, T. (2025, February 9). *Key facts about hospitals.* KFF. https://www.kff.org/key-facts-about-hospitals/?entry=hospital-finances-profit-margins

61   United States Census Bureau. (n.d.). *American Community Survey, Table S1301, "Fertility."* https://data.census.gov/table?q=Table%20S1301

62   Boscoe, F. P., Henry, K. A., & Zdeb, M. S. (2012). A nationwide comparison of driving distance versus straight-line distance to hospitals. *The Professional Geographer: The Journal of the Association of American Geographers, 64*(2), 10.1080/00330124.2011.583586. https://doi.org/10.1080/00330124.2011.583586

63   Haynes, E. (2023). *Motherhood and mental illness: A relational treatment approach.* Routledge.

64   Haynes, E. (2023). *Motherhood and mental illness: A relational treatment approach.* Routledge.

65   Gooch, R. (1829). *An account of some of the most important diseases peculiar to women.* Barrington and Haswell.

66   Held, L., & Rutherford, A. (2012). Can't a mother sing the blues? Postpartum depression and the construction of motherhood in late 20th-century America. *History of Psychology, 15*(2), 107–123. https://doi.org/10.1037/a0026219

67   Chen, Y., Shiels, M. S., Uribe-Leitz, T., Molina, R. L., Lawrence, W. R., Freedman, N. D., & Abnet, C. C. (2025). Pregnancy-related deaths in the US, 2018-2022. *JAMA Network Open, 8*(4), e254325. https://doi.org/10.1001/jamanetworkopen.2025.4325

68   Centers for Disease Control and Prevention. (2025, August 22). *Pregnancy-related deaths: Data from Maternal Mortality Review Committees.* https://www.cdc.gov/maternal-mortality/php/data-research/mmrc-2017-2019.html

69   Grote, N. K., Bridge, J. A., Gavin, A. R., Melville, J. L., Iyengar, S., & Katon, W. J. (2010). A Meta-analysis of depression during pregnancy and the risk of preterm birth, low birth weight, and intrauterine growth

restriction. *Archives of General Psychiatry, 67*(10), 1012–1024. https://doi. org/10.1001/archgenpsychiatry.2010.111

70 Christoforou, A., Duman, E. A., & Caparros-Gonzalez, R. A. (2025). Editorial: Intergenerational impacts of perinatal mental health. *Frontiers in Psychiatry, 16*, 1542112. https://doi.org/10.3389/fpsyt.2025.1542112

71 Zero To Three. (2024, August 15). *Maternal mental health and prenatal brain development: A proven link.* https://www.zerotothree.org/resource/maternal-mental-health-and-prenatal-brain-development-a-proven-link/

72 Monk, C. (2025, January 28). *Parenting begins in pregnancy.* Early Childhood Matters. https://earlychildhoodmatters.online/2025/parenting-begins-in-pregnancy/

73 National Institute of Mental Health. (2025, August). *Suicide.* https://www. nimh.nih.gov/health/statistics/suicide

74 Centers for Disease Control and Prevention. (2024, November 29). *Mental health.* https://www.cdc.gov/healthy-youth/mental-health/index.html

75 National Institute of Mental Health. (2025, August). *Suicide.* https://www. nimh.nih.gov/health/statistics/suicide

76 National Institute of Mental Health. (2023). *Perinatal depression.* https https://www.nimh.nih.gov/health/publications/perinatal-depression

77 Luca, D. L., Margiotta, C., Staatz, C., Garlow, E., Christensen, A., & Zivin, K. (2020). Financial toll of untreated perinatal mood and anxiety disorders among 2017 births in the United States. *American Journal of Public Health, 110*(6), 888–896. https://doi.org/10.2105/AJPH.2020.305619

78 Brown, C. C., Adams, C. E., George, K. E., & Moore, J. E. (2021). Mental health conditions increase severe maternal morbidity by 50 percent and cost $102 million yearly in the United States. *Health Affairs (Project Hope), 40*(10), 1575–1584. https://doi.org/10.1377/hlthaff.2021.00759

79 Luca, D. L., Margiotta, C., Staatz, C., Garlow, E., Christensen, A., & Zivin, K. (2020). Financial toll of untreated perinatal mood and anxiety disorders among 2017 births in the United States. *American Journal of Public Health, 110*(6), 888–896. https://doi.org/10.2105/AJPH.2020.305619

80 Quiñones, F., Winters, C., Hu, L., & Suvarnakar, A. (2023). Untreated major depression during gestation: The physical and mental implications in women and their offspring. *Georgetown Medical Review, 7*(1). https://doi. org/10.52504/001c.83340

81 Perinatal Support International. (n.d.). *Intensive treatment in the US.* https:// postpartum.net/get-help/intensive-perinatal-psych-treatment-in-the-us/

INDEX